CARING LESSONS

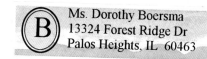
In her book, Mrs. Roelofs, the Ph.D., the RN, the wife, and the mother wears her titles gracefully as she weaves a web of suspense, adventure, compassion, and love. With an honest, open, and conversational brush she paints a vivid picture of life with all its trials and tribulations. We need more psychiatric nurses and teachers like her to help lift the stigma from mental illness. This book is a great comfort to women trying to balance career, motherhood, and commitment to the greater good of mankind.

—Sel Erder Yackley, author of
Never Regret the Pain: Loving and Losing a Bipolar Spouse

In *Caring Lessons*, Dr. Roelofs tells of her life's journey through an intricate maze of professional experiences, each one building on the last, to eventually find herself as a doctorally prepared nurse in academia. As one who can identify with several of the author's roles—psychiatric nurse, professor, and administrator—I found the manuscript to be engaging and candid. It is a delightful must-read for nurses that will leave you amused, tearful, proud, and, in the end, richer for having been invited into Roelofs' professional life.

—Mary Molewyk Doornbos, Ph.D., RN, Professor and Chairperson,
Department of Nursing, Calvin College, and co-author of
Transforming Care: A Christian Vision of Nursing Practice

I hooted, cried, and reminisced all the way through *Caring Lessons*. Lois and I met at the Iowa Summer Writing Festival and, although traveling different career paths, we each encountered many of the same expectations and restrictions concerning the "womanly" use of our gifts. This book is a testament to her ability to draw even those of us who never donned a nurse's cap, or gave a patient a bed bath, or lectured on schizophrenia, into her lifetime of experiences as a nurse and an educator as if they were our own. Beautiful writing; heartwarming story!

—Carol Rottman, Ph.D., author of *Writers in the Spirit* and
All Nature Sings: A Spiritual Journey of Place

In today's environment of spiraling healthcare costs, nursing shortages and health care reform, *Caring Lessons* is a powerful yet delightful commentary on the fears, joys, and culminating pride to be found in a nursing career. The author reminds us not only of what it is like to evolve from a naïve nursing student to a successful professional, but also the challenges of juggling family joys and tragedies while pursuing a career. Thoughtful, sensitive, and revealing, this is one of the most heartwarming books I have read in a long time.

—Patsy L. Ruchala, DNSc, RN, Professor and Director,
Orvis School of Nursing, University of Nevada, Reno

I loved this book. Lois has a wonderful ability to capture the experiences she had and tie them to thought-provoking themes. I'm full of admiration for the tone. It's an authentic, often humorous, unfolding of a life that not only has been well-lived, but well-studied. Without making a big point of her faith, her story is one of spiritual growth as she explores who she needed to become. She has given us a good example of following the artist's way to the deepest expression of self.

—Ann Brody, M.S.W., Career/Life Coach,
Career Solutions, Inc., Chicago

CARING LESSONS

A Nursing Professor's Journey
of Faith and Self

For Dorothy —
In appreciation to
you for helping
us start TCC's
nursing program.
You were the
best - competent
and cordial - Always!
Lois

LOIS HOITENGA ROELOFS

Matt. 5:7 "You're blessed when you care..."

Deep River
B O O K S

Author's note: The stories here are true, but they are my memories and no one else's. I have changed the names and identifying details of all individuals except for my family members and my friend Marianna. And I've referred to all nursing students, regardless of gender, as females. Readers may connect with me by visiting loisroelofs.com

Caring Lessons

Published by
Deep River Books
Sisters, Oregon
http://www.deepriverbooks.com

ISBN 10 1-935265-37-7
ISBN 13 978-1-935265-37-5

Library of Congress: 2010931650

Printed in the USA

Cover design by www.blackbirdcreative.biz

To my kindred spirits

in their quest for learning, caring, and making a difference
and
in memory of my parents
Rev. Dewey James Hoitenga, Sr., and
Mrs. Theresa (Tess) Vander Meer Hoitenga

Acknowledgments

My thanks to my patients, students, colleagues, and mentors for giving me invaluable insights, never-ending opportunities to care, and a most fun, challenging, and rewarding career. And to Marianna Crane, my dear and loyal friend, for traveling with me through countless capers in our careers and inspiring me to write this book—it never would have happened without her.

My thanks to writing teachers and fellow students at the Newberry Library and the Iowa Summer Writing Festival for affirming the worth and interest of a nurse's story. And to readers along the way for feedback and encouragement: Ann Brody, Barbara Doyle, Mark Foreman, Mary Lebold, Kimberly Oosterhouse, Burt Rozema, Cynthia Sander, Gerald Stein, my sisters Kay Hoitenga, Kay Korthuis, and Esther Van Zytveld, and to readers of the final manuscript for their comments and editorial assistance: Susan Hanes, my sister Rose Kossen, and my niece Noralyn Masselink.

My thanks to the Tuesday Writers—Lois Barliant, Pepper Furey, and Linda Keane—for critiquing each word, sentence, and paragraph. Draft after draft. Week after week. For most of nine years. And to Deep River Books for selecting my book for publication, and to Bill Carmichael, Lacey Ogle, and Laura Cowan for walking along with me in the process.

My special thanks to my children, Jon Roelofs and Kathleen Roelofs Ridder, for humoring their career mom—taking turns vacuuming and making peanut butter and jelly lunches—and being the most important addition to their dad's and my life. And to my second daughter and son, Sheri Roosendaal Roelofs and Michael Ridder, for the love and spice they've added to our family.

And my special love to my grandchildren—Kristin, Kyle, and Megan Roelofs, and our newest addition, Madison Tessa Ridder. This book is for them and their children. My wish is that it will help them know and appreciate the life of one nurse in the second half of the twentieth century, their grandma who "loves you little and loves you big"—as my mother loved me and as I love their parents.

And, finally, my warmest thanks to Marv for fifty years of love and listening.

Contents

Nursing is an art; and if it is to be made an art,
it requires as exclusive a devotion, as hard a preparation,
as any painter's or sculptor's work.
For what is the having to do with dead canvas or cold marble
compared with having to do with the living body—the
temple of God's spirit?
It is one of the fine arts;
I had almost said, the finest of the fine arts.

Florence Nightingale,
To the editor, *Macmillan's Magazine*, April, 1867.[1]

[1] *As Miss Nightingale Said...*, ed. M. Baly. (London: Scutari Press, 1991).

A FEW NOTES ON WRITING

My mother often said her best birthday present arrived on her thirty-ninth birthday. The present was me. The pregnancy had been stressful (more about that later), and my dad and my four siblings and a caregiver "auntie," plus many others, were relieved that both my mother and I survived. With obvious joy, my blind and deaf grandma, Helen Vander Meer, wrote a poem to my mother celebrating our safe arrival home from the Mahaska County hospital in Oskaloosa, Iowa, titling it "Welcome Home":

> Now, my dear, you're home again
> God has answered all our prayers.
> After weeks and weeks of strain,
> Days and nights of loving care.
>
> My imagination tells me
> They have crowded all so near,
> Dewey, Kathleen, Helen, Esther,
> Just to see their mother dear.
>
> And that precious little bundle,
> Wrapped all up in flannel white,
> I can hear their merry laughter,
> In their joy of great delight.
>
> Daddy looking in amazement
> Down upon his happy six.
> Auntie full of smiles and saying,
> "What a happy scene is this."
>
> And then Grandma, softly singing,
> Lullabys [*sic*] for Lois Anne,

And we all thank God together
Who has made all things so well.

My grandma's poetry may have inspired my interest in writing, but I wasn't aware of it on August 4, 2000, when I perched on the departures curb at O'Hare and basked in the brightness of the morning sun. That warm day felt like a day of promise, a day to begin my final third of life. Settling into a narrow coach seat, I ignored my neighbor and read my brand-new, first copy of *Writer's Digest*. I felt like a traitor. Who was I, anyway, to be reading articles on writing? I'd spent the last forty years reading, eating, and sleeping nursing.

The *Writer's Digest* offered no articles on the four concepts that frame nursing curricula—nursing, person, environment, and health—which I'd taught for the previous twenty years. As I read words like "character," "scene," "dialogue," and "plot," that's all they were—words. I had no reference points. Immediately, I knew how my students must've felt when I attempted to enlighten them about patients' "self-care deficits" and "therapeutic self-care demands."

I slid my hand into the soft cotton pocket of my baggy bib jeans to find a pencil. I loved those jeans. I loved being fifty-eight, shedding my lab coat, and wearing kid-like, farmer-type overalls. I loved it when other women my age said, "I can't get by with wearing that, Lois, but you can."

Even my last year's nursing students had said, "They are *so* you, Dr. Roelofs." They'd said the same thing on the last day of clinical about my new retirement Beetle. Purplish blue, I'd told them, because I was now an old woman and I could drive purple.

Attitude helped my aging process. Being upbeat. Not only wearing bib jeans, but also a trendy black knit jacket. I wore black, not because anyone would find it in my color wheel—they wouldn't—but because my students had been wearing lots of black, and I wanted to be in fashion. For me, a grandma of three, passing muster as a trendy college professor rated high on my status thermometer. And my husband, Marv, was used to me not wanting to look old or to act old.

I was on my way to see my friend Marianna in Chapel Hill. The purpose for this visit had come up a few months before. While talking on the phone, we decided we should write stories from our nursing careers. So now we were getting together for a whole week, longer than any former visit, to plan our stories. Two nurses, 1962 graduates of different diploma programs, leaving their comfort zones of nursing to write books. Once we dreamed up something, nothing had stopped us. Ever.

After landing at Raleigh Durham, I stepped into the terminal and spotted Marianna poised to take my picture. She was wearing black knit slacks and a white crewneck T-shirt, clothes that complemented her whitish-gray flipped hair. Age-appropriate clothes. Walking through the airport, oblivious of other travelers, we talked nonstop as we wove our way through the parking garage to her car. She drove a Volvo; until that year, I'd driven a Plymouth. On the way home, we stopped at Harris Teeter's. Marianna needed to do some "food shopping." I "grocery shop." In the produce section, Marianna inspected and selected one piece of fruit at a time. I schlep through and grab five-pound bags. I liked our differences. Since I'd forgotten to pack toothpaste, I wandered off and found a tiny tube labeled ginger. Perfect, I thought. It's time to ditch the traditional Colgate. The zing of ginger felt more romantic for my new writing life.

We arrived at Marianna's windowy home in the woods around lunchtime. Sitting on her deck overlooking a ravine reminded me of being immersed in a forest preserve near my home in Palos Heights, a Chicago suburb. With the sun splashing through the branches across our faces, the deck created a Zen-like setting to contemplate the what, where, when, how, and why of our nursing careers. Marianna and I liked to mull over life. Over our nearly thirty-year friendship, we had asked each other, at least monthly, "What do you want to be when you grow up?" And we'd answered each other, "I don't know." Maybe with this writing adventure, we'd find some clues.

That week, we cozied up at opposite ends of her floral cotton couch. During twenty-minute time spans, we ambled in our minds down miles of hallways in all of our workplaces, writing lists of potential stories. Then we read our lists and told stories about every item to each other, prompting more memories, often ones we'd successfully repressed. "Oh, yes," I remember saying, "I once felt like I caused a person to die, too." My very first written sentence was: "For the umpteenth time that summer of 1960, I called home to beg my dad to let me quit nurses' training." He obviously didn't.

Walking past Rodin's *The Thinker* at the Museum of Art in Raleigh, we brainstormed some more, plopping on a bench to jot down our thoughts before they left our minds. Sitting in a sunny gazebo at Fearrington Village, a cat slithering over our notebooks, we wrote why we wanted to put our stories on paper: "I feel like I'm full of words that need to come out."

After the week was up, we shared drafts by e-mail and met in person once or twice a year—at her home, or my home. Or on destination trips to the Grand Ole Opry in Nashville, Ground Zero in New York City, and The Pier Aquarium in downtown St. Petersburg. After each day's excursions, we'd curl up on our beds, write in our journals, and make our next plans for writing. We also took writing courses, started critique groups, and met in Iowa City to study memoir at the Iowa Summer Writing Festival. Along the way, we fortified ourselves with mochas, hot fudge sundaes, and giant chocolate chip cookies.

For my book, I wanted to capture as many details as I could while I still remembered them. The result is a potpourri of stories dipping in and out of my nursing life, nearly all coming from those first lists I created with Marianna.

And, now that I'm finished, for the record, I still don't know what I want to be when I grow up. I do know, with nursing shortages, so few nursing memoirs in the bookstores, and significant health care changes on the horizon, nursing stories are needed to inform, to inspire, and, yes, to provide humor to all nurses, and to the public—many of whom will wake up someday and see the caring face of a nurse.

PART ONE

Diploma

One

SWEET LITTLE HOITIE

The smell of pines. The warmth of sunshine breaking through the trees. The sounds of birds in the branches calling to the morning. A path, carpeted with pine needles, leading to a one-and-a-half-story white stucco building, a homey place smelling of freshly baked bread. A psychiatric hospital for older women. In a dayroom, twelve ladies, secured in their tray-chairs and dressed in their best Sunday cottons, were waiting for me, sound asleep.

Except for Greta and Tryntje.

"Hoitie, Hoitie, you're here today!" Greta welcomed me at the half-door, her black hair pulled back tightly into a bun, shoulders rounded, Bible pressed against her chest.

"Hey la-a-a-y-dee. Hey la-a-a-y-dee," Tryntje sang from the right-hand corner. She sat straight up on a vinyl-padded armchair, legs stretched out on a stool. Her short gray bob framed a child-like grin.

"Morning, Greta. Morning, Tryntje." I grinned as I turned my key in the door; their simple joy was contagious.

Inside the dayroom, I slipped past the sleeping ladies on my left and switched on the knob of the wooden loudspeaker in the corner of the ceiling.

"Lois Hoitenga," a voice said from behind me, by the half-door. "I'm glad you're on today."

Sticking my thumbs behind the cloth belt of my uniform—a starched green dress with a white collar—to adjust it on my hips, I turned to see Mrs. Kingma, the charge nurse. But to me, she was Cherry Ames. I'd read Cherry Ames books as a child—the stories about a dark-haired, bright-lipped, multi-talented nurse, never expecting to meet her in person. But, here in my first job at Pine Rest Christian Hospital in Cutlerville, on the south end of Grand Rapids, Michigan, she'd come to life.

"We can tell when you work the back ward, Lois, because the ladies' hair has been waved. When they're lined up in their tray-chairs, their heads look like a shiny row of gray ripples. How do you do that?" Her eyes sparkled under her dark bouncy curls tamed by bobby pins and topped with a starched white cap.

I felt myself blush. "I comb their hair back, braid it, and then circle it into a bun. But I leave the top a little loose, so I can wave it by crunching it between the sides of my fingers. I try to make them look like my grandma used to. Only she used crimpers, springy metal things with teeth."

"Well, the ladies look pretty." She turned and handed me a small paper cup. "Here are the pills for this morning. They all get this orange one. Make sure they swallow them."

I never thought it unusual that I, as a nurse's aide, was entrusted to give my ladies their medications. Meds I'd not set up, so I hadn't read their labels. Sort of like being handed a small cup of M&Ms and being asked to hand them out. At seventeen, being able to give the meds made me feel important in my eighty-cents-an-hour job.

After Mrs. Kingma left, organ music, piped in from the hospital chapel, broke into the room. As I prodded each lady awake to give her a pill, patients in the chapel began to sing: "Holy, Holy, Holy! Lord God Almighty." My twelve ladies roused with the familiar tune and chimed in. My ladies, who otherwise wore mute, senseless, or agitated expressions, now sang lustily, tapping their fingers on their tray tables. One could not guess why they were here.

I loved to sing hymns with my ladies. I'd learned them all growing up in a parsonage. My dad was the minister of the local Christian Reformed church. I loved to quiet my ladies' hands when they were banging on their tray tables. I loved to unstrap my ladies and walk with them outside through the fragrant pines to the sidewalk that bordered town.

But I hated having to lock them back up into their tray-table life. I gagged when I had to wipe bottoms during a trip to the bathroom. I grew weary of being on guard for a heavy swat across the face.

And, leaving the dayroom at the end of my shift, I'd look back and scan my rectangular arrangement of ladies—some snoring, some drooling, some muttering to themselves—and my heart would be tormented with the thought, *What if someday this mental deterioration happens to my mother? Or my sisters? Or me?* I wasn't sure I was cut out for this work. Snapping me out of morbidity, Greta would often sidle up to the half-door and thrust a letter into my hand, one of which I've saved. I can still see her, head bent over the table, pressing each period on the paper with diligent precision. "Read it on your way home, Hoitie," she'd say, as she'd grasp my hands and twirl her tongue around her toothless mouth.

Grand Rapids Mich.

July 10, 1.9.5.9.

My Sweet little Hoitie!

I am so very glad that you are here today once again and I hope you will do it oftener. for it is so precious to have you in our midst—such a dear little girl like you are. You are all sunshine, dear heart. You are my good little nursie and that stands securely. I love you so very much and I enjoyed this day again with you…it was Showers of Blessings indeed…. I had such a nice walk with you this morning too…. I will be sorry when this day is over again with you for I'll miss you so much….Well, I must end here. so good bye Hoitie mine. Lots of love and best wishes to a darling little soul. I am your friend most deeply.

   Greta. Van Der. Meer.

I didn't, however, feel like Greta's "Sweet Little Hoitie" in the struggles I was having at home about starting nurses' training that fall. I wanted to be a stewardess, but I never told anyone. I knew, even as a little girl in the fifties, becoming a stewardess wouldn't be acceptable for a preacher's daughter. Everyone knew the "coffee, tea, or me" women led loose lives. I'd never even flown, but I'd seen ads— stewardesses boarding planes, waving and smiling. I wanted to be one of them— taking off, going somewhere. Anywhere.

In my home, a girl was supposed to become a teacher or a nurse. Without discussion, I understood these were noble professions for girls. For a boy, seminary was okay. My brother, the oldest of our family of five children, did that. For girls, teaching and nursing were also good jobs to fall back on if our husbands died, or, even worse, if they should leave us. Of my three older sisters, the oldest was a nurse, the second a teacher, and the third had followed her heart to work in business. But I did as I was told, never even thought to question.

Grading papers with my fifth-grade-teacher mother squelched any desire I may have had to become a teacher. After supper, she'd say, "Would you please help me grade a stack of papers tonight? I have four sets of arithmetic."

As the "baby" of the family and the only child left at home to help, what could I say? Many an evening, my mother and I sat side by side on our rose-colored, camel-backed davenport while I read lists of right answers. "One, 431; two, 58; three, 972.... " I hated it.

So, I reluctantly chose nursing. Luckily, I was in love with my sister Kay's student nurse's uniform. She was in nurses' training at Blodgett Memorial Hospital in Grand Rapids. Sometimes when I came home from junior high, she'd be sitting on the davenport in her uniform, a blue and white pinstriped dress covered with an angelic-white, stiffly-starched, calf-length apron. When I sat next to her, I could smell the heavy sweet odor of starch. I admired her opaque white nylons—probably even the support kind—that I could see for a few inches between her apron and her shiny white leather "duty" shoes.

But I loved her starched, box-shaped cap that lay beside her the most. Securing it on the back of my head with a bobby pin on my crown—the goal was to have the cap invisible from the front, I looked in the large mirror above the fireplace in our red brick, two-story, colonial parsonage and imagined myself, clean and pure, floating up and down hospital hallways, healing the sick. With the power of the uniform, I would become my own version of Cherry Ames.

I did not want to go to school in the shadow of my sister. Kay, an A student, had graduated from Blodgett in 1955 and helped open the first intensive care unit there. I tried begging my folks: "Could I please go to the University of Michigan instead of Blodgett? Our nursing supervisor at Pine Rest went there...." I wanted to move farther from home, and I liked the supervisor's cap. It was rectangular rather than square and would look slimmer on the back of my head.

My folks looked at me with sober expressions. I'm sure I exasperated them, but they stayed consistent: "You'll go to Calvin like your brother and sisters did." Calvin College was our denominational college; I'm sure it looked better for my minister dad if I went there. It was about ten miles from our home, and the first year of classes for Blodgett's three-year diploma nursing program was offered there.

I started the pre-nursing program at Calvin in the fall of 1959. I struggled for Cs in the sciences. Even Old Testament History was a challenge. All those dates. I got As only in psychology. When Debbie, the girl I planned to room with at Blodgett, decided in late spring to go back to college in the fall, out of town, to become a teacher, I was devastated. I begged my dad to allow me to join her. "I could teach English, like Rose." (My sister Helen, mentioned in my grandma's poem in the prologue, had adopted her middle name, Rose, in grade school.)

She had turned me on, as my high school American Literature teacher, to the pleasures of assonance, alliteration, and onomatopoeia as we studied Poe, Whitman, and Dickinson.

My begging didn't work. "No, I don't think so," my dad said at the dinner table. "You've taken the pre-nursing courses now. You must give the summer a try."

I don't remember my mother getting involved with this conversation. I see her busying herself with dishing up dessert, probably leftover cake baked for Sunday evening visits with members of the congregation.

After a few short weeks of summer break, I moved into the dorm of Blodgett's nursing school on June 26, 1960. The next day was our capping ceremony. That night I opened my new diary book, *On Call: Daily Devotions for Nurses,* and wrote: "Dull lectures in A.M. Unimpressive capping in P.M. Reception at night. Really fun. Got Joe-Marv—a stuffed basset hound with big floppy ears from Jayne [high school friend], this [diary] book from Esther and Dave [sister and husband]. Shoes, duster, and overnight case from folks."

I missed Marv, the boyfriend I'd met the first day at Calvin standing in front of the administration building on Franklin Street during a break in orientation. A friend of mine, who had met him sitting in alphabetical order during testing, introduced us. Marv was wearing the collar up on his khaki raincoat and dangling a cigarette from his mouth—the perfect Marlboro man. When he stared into my eyes, laughing low and gently to my giggly remarks, I was sure he was God-sent; I had prayed the night before that I'd find a boyfriend at college. I knew right away I would marry him. Now he was back home in Minnesota working on road construction for the summer. The best I could do in his absence was name my new stuffed dog after him and my first crush in grade school, a neighbor five years older—the neighbor getting first dibs.

The party and gifts were the best part of the day. The lectures and my own starched white cap did not impress me. I simply wasn't sure I wanted to be a nurse. How could I finagle going back to college in the fall after all? That night I lay awake trying to figure out how the smattering of English, Bible, psychology, chemistry, anatomy and physiology, and microbiology I'd taken at Calvin could count toward another major.

"Missy," he said, voice raspy, eyes sunken, "You just take care of it. Don't make me look at it. Or smell it. Or listen to it." He grabbed my hand as I stood at the right side of his bed. "You make me better."

I was working the day shift on Men's Ward, assigned to Mr. Becker, an elderly farmer dying from colon cancer. Stuffed inside the airless space between the curtains and his bed in the center of the ward, I was assigned to bathe him and change his colostomy dressing.

As I lifted off the thick pack of reddish-yellow, drainage-filled gauze dressings, I couldn't tell him I didn't want to look at his stoma either. The red, angry twist of swollen colon, ironically called a rosebud, sat on his abdomen, bowel contents oozing over its sides. The skin around the stoma was an angrier red and was blistering open from being eaten away by the drainage. The bathroom smell launched my breakfast juice toward my throat. I could not let him see that the sight and odor bothered me. I turned my head to the side, took a deep breath, swallowed, turned back, and attempted a smile. "I'll do the best I can, Mr. Becker."

I felt helpless.

That first summer had plunged me into an oppressive new reality. There was no Cherry Ames' glamour on that Men's Ward. Not between the dull blue walls that soared up to what must have been fifteen-foot ceilings. Not when open wooden-screened windows sent in suffocating heat. Not when BM-streaked bedpans and urine-drizzled urinals discharged stomach-turning smells.

Every time I walked into the ward, I sensed twelve pairs of hollow male eyes watching my every move. I felt uncomfortably on stage. All the patients were old men with bowel or urinary problems. It seemed all my patients, wizened and huddled behind their bed curtains, were in Beds 11 or 12 in the center of the ward. It was on that ward I practiced my first procedures, called nursing skills today. As students, we spent hours in the nursing arts lab, learning everything nurses do with patients from a 1959 book I still have: *Manual of Nursing Procedures, Blodgett Memorial Hospital, Grand Rapids 6, Michigan.* We were expected to be able to remember, step by step, each procedure on a moment's notice. All summer, I bathed frail bodies, changed surgical dressings, irrigated first bowel movements out of new colostomies, flushed clots from urinary catheters in newly reamed out urethras.

As the days progressed, I felt as though I was steadily succumbing to my patients' sadness, as though I was drowning in fluids—from shriveled bodies, irrigation tubes, enema cans, IV bottles, glass syringes. My starched uniform became as limp as my mood. I couldn't believe I was spending my eighteenth summer feeling blue in a blue room learning all things I never wanted to know about bowels and bladders. I envied my hoped-for roommate Debbie, probably lying on the beach at Tunnel Park in Holland, talking about boys, reading *True Confessions*, planning for her teaching major in the fall. Trivial things compared to my responsibility for keeping people alive.

I started having trouble sleeping. I kept asking myself the same question: Who in their right mind would want to be a nurse? I mean, *really*, who would ever want to be a nurse? I took to shaking my leg vigorously to rid myself of tension and get myself to sleep.

So, unlike Florence Nightingale, who as early as age seven felt called by God to become a nurse, I, at eighteen, only wanted to run away from this hot, smelly, suffering place. But since my folks allowed no alternative, I had to stay. Every morning, before I got out of my dorm bed, I prayed, *Dear God, help me get through this day.* Not a very churchly prayer, but it came from the aching chambers of my heart. I could not do this alone; I knew I needed divine help to survive.

After my shift caring for Mr. Becker, I once again had had enough. I hurried through the brick pagoda-style archway, a girl with a mission, to the dorm behind the hospital, slid back the grate of the small elevator in the lobby, pushed the 2 button, scurried to my room, threw my smelly uniform into a muslin laundry bag at the back of my closet, and took a shower in the communal bathroom. "Go on ahead to supper," I told my roommate. "I need a nap."

I really needed to call home.

I staked out the darkened hallway and listened for talking or radio noise coming over transoms. As soon as I was sure most of the girls had gone to supper, I dashed down the hall to the telephone bench by the fire door. I perched on the edge of the seat to beg my dad for the umpteenth time to let me quit nurses' training. Holding my breath, I dialed home: Lenox 2-6262. I peered down the hot, narrow hallway one last time to make sure I was alone. Eyeing the open transoms, I said a quick prayer: *Please, God, don't let anyone overhear what I'm about to say.*

My dad answered. I pictured him, a half hour away, sitting at the large mahogany desk in his study in the parsonage, black hair parted in the middle, rimless glasses. Solemn.

I started right in before I chickened out. "Dad, I can't stay here any longer. This time I mean it. I hate the things I have to do. I want to come home."

There was a long pause. An audible swallow. He cleared his throat and then delivered his probably least favorite but most repeated sermon of the summer. "Mother and I have talked about it. We would like you to stick it out until September…to complete the probationary period."

I grabbed my throat to hold onto a tidbit of hope and tried a small voice. "I can't handle it anymore, Dad. The pain. The suffering. The dying…I can't get to sleep anymore. I'm waking up at night with horrible dreams." In my mind, I heard Mr. Becker's pleas for help. I had to try convincing my dad one last time. "I'd much rather go back to college in the fall. I'd like to try teaching."

Another pause. I remembered him, during my sophomore summer when I'd had mono, bringing breakfast to me in my room across the hall from his study—a bowl of Wheaties, a fluffy slice of my mother's homemade bread, a generous dollop of fresh strawberry jam—and, before he left me, sitting on the opposite twin bed to say a prayer with me. I wished for his soft side to pop up again.

I heard him take a breath. "We've been through this before. If you pass the probationary period, and you're still sure you want to quit, we'll reconsider."

I slumped in a heap on the telephone bench. In my mind I saw myself in the maple rocker at the foot of his desk where my mother used to send me to sit for punishment of any wrongdoing. I spent plenty of time in that chair; my worst offense was going out with a guy they had forbidden me to date. They found out when we hurried home to call a tow truck after we'd gotten stuck while parking in an empty muddy ball field near my house. They were as quiet as I was as I sat out my punishment. My chair sentence seemed to be more painful for them than for me.

Now, my head said any further pleading was useless. I would have to stay. I was stuck at Blodgett, rooming with another girl who had no roommate. Stuck in a small room with maple bunk beds and bland walls. Stuck in Grand Rapids—probably for life.

I hurried through the August humidity on the slippery tiled floor back to my room. I didn't want to face classmates at supper, but I needed to eat. The dorm's only snack bar was across the hall. A women's guild furnished the room with food, probably for days like I was having. I toasted a piece of white bread, slathered it with peanut butter and grape jam, and poured a glass of apple juice. Sitting alone at the bar, I took small bites, trying to settle my queasy stomach and quiet the pitter-patter in my chest. As I followed each bite with juice, I stared out the window at the dark brick hospital from the only room in the dorm that felt even remotely like home.

The ten-week probationary period drew to a close. By then I was trapped into staying because colleges were already starting. I told myself I could stand to stay a few more months because my Section A clinical group was scheduled to go to obstetrics. New babies should be a cheerful change from my somber medical-surgical summer. And as long as I'd decided to stay, I was eager to show I was no longer a probie—a probationary student—by gluing a narrow black-velvet stripe, designating junior status, on my plain white cap. Each of the junior and senior years would last twelve months.

It never occurred to me my class wouldn't all go on together.

One day, after a lecture in the hospital's first-floor classroom, my friend Kate met me in the dorm hallway, motioned me to stop, and asked me, quietly, to be her roommate.

I was stunned. "What do you mean? What's going on?"

She whispered, "My roommate's been let go. While some of us were in class, lots of girls were told they had to leave." I could barely hear her. Her brown eyes flashed.

About a third of our class of sixty hadn't passed probation. They couldn't become juniors. So they had packed up, called their folks to pick them up, and were already gone.

Silence gripped me. What could this mean? Why was I spared? Didn't anyone know I hated this? Hadn't anyone been able to tell?

I accepted Kate's invitation. We'd met at Calvin, sitting in alphabetical order. Getting back together was a happy thing. Since we were both in Section A, we would be doing the same clinical rotations and it'd be fun to compare experiences in the evening in our own room.

A day later, a note in my student mailbox summoned me to the office of the director of the School of Nursing. I took my time going through the archway to her office in the hospital. She sat, stiff and starched behind her desk in her white, impeccable, long-sleeved uniform and winged cap, facing me. Her voice was soft. "Miss Hoitenga, your instructors aren't sure you should be here."

Wham. I'd survived the purge, but now that I'd decided to stay, were they going to humiliate me by sending me home? What would my folks say?

"I hear there's a problem with your attitude on the ward."

Every cell of my five-foot, five-inch, 120-pound frame shivered with fear. I heard myself pleading with her. "I'm having a hard time doing all the smelly procedures. But I'm sure it will get better as I get used to it."

"If you want to stay," she said as if she hadn't heard me, "we will give you a chance to improve your attitude. We are reassigning you from Section A to Section B. So rather than going with your group to the obstetrics specialty this fall, you will remain in a medical-surgical area for another three months. That will give you time, in a familiar setting, to work on your attitude."

Attitude. I did not understand, but I was not going to ask. I just wanted to get out of the starched office. I felt I had no choice, ironically, but to thank her for the chance to stay.

My "demotion" meant Kate and I would never be in the same rotation. Since we did our three-month psychiatric rotation later on in Chicago, we would live apart six months of our remaining twenty-four months. Kate was an upbeat source of comfort. "We'll help you, Hoit." But, she reminded me with a laugh, "If you would've behaved yourself, we could've done all our rotations together."

The best thing about that fall was settling into a new room, an end room outside the fire doors, with Kate. She immediately plopped a fluffy tan rug she'd gotten from her boyfriend in front of the dresser. She allowed no one but herself to step on it. To get anything out of a dresser drawer, I had to do arm stretches or deep knee bends. She positioned her gigantic green can of April Showers on the middle of the maple double dresser. After every shower, she ran back to our room swathed in towels, one around her head, the other around her body, and stood on the fluffy rug. She dropped the body towel, stood naked, and shook clouds of April Showers over her chest, back, and legs, turning the rug into tufts of cotton candy and the surrounding asphalt-tiled floor into a ski slope.

She was fun to watch. She made me laugh.

Except for the rug, the room was barren. So I decided to contribute a doily for under the can of April Showers. Taking one of my starched uniform aprons, I draped the bib and back straps behind the dresser and spread the wrap-around skirt across the dresser top. The skirt-turned-doily looked crisp and clean, precisely the way we did when we wore the apron. But, within a week, I found another note in my mailbox: "Please do not use your apron for a dresser scarf. This is a warning. Thank you, House Committee."

So many "warnings" and something awful would happen; I don't remember what.

Part of me said getting a warning for such a dumb thing was a joke, but another part said, *If they don't like my behavior in the dorm, how will I ever get my attitude to be acceptable in the clinical?* It wasn't like me to plaster on a happy face to please others. So, how would I pull off this attitude change? When would the next note appear in my mailbox? How soon would I be packing to go home? As a former "Sweet Little Hoitie," I still wasn't feeling too sweet.

Two

A MATTER OF ATTITUDE

My attitude change. It was absolutely no fun having the aura of a bad attitude haunting me through my junior and senior years. I might as well have had an engraving on my forehead that said, "Hey, look at me. I'm the student who has to be watched." It's no wonder, with my perceived pressure of needing to be perfect, that what I remember best are the times I messed up. And the pranks I participated in for survival. And then the time, toward the end of my senior year, when I was pleasantly surprised.

In September of 1960, as a new junior student proudly wearing one thin, black velvet stripe on my cap, signifying my new status, I reported for duty determined to be the most cheerful, cooperative, and jim-dandy student to have around. My instructor, short, squat, and blonde, assigned me a patient in isolation—Class A, respiratory—the most complex type of isolation procedure designed to protect me from the patient. It required not only gowning and gloving, but also masking to avoid breathing in germ-filled droplets in the air. Because it was my first time, as had become my custom, I pulled up the picture in my head of my procedure book, recalled several pages on "isolation," including pictures, and ran through over thirty steps in my mind. There were steps involving the masking, gowning, gloving. Taking the temperature, pulse, respiration. Disposing of dishes, linen, wastebasket, contaminated equipment. I needed to have all my wits alert, which I did all morning until I left the room.

I don't remember the patient. I remember he (or she) was confined to the bed aligned with the left wall of the room. Straight ahead was a window. And what I remember is the unused IV pole standing in front of it.

As we stood outside the patient's room, the instructor peeked through a crack in the doorway and said, "What is that IV pole still doing in there?"

I didn't know. I guessed it was because I thought it might be used again. Before I could answer, she said, "You didn't want to have to wipe it down, did you?"

Nothing I said could convince her that I plain messed up, that I wasn't simply lazy. I needed to swallow my words because, clearly, becoming combative wasn't going to earn me attitude points. That incident happened after several days of being on a high because I'd accomplished a complicated procedure for setting up medications that involved numerous steps, also meticulously memorized, that ended up with rows and rows of meds—pills in paper ketchup-like cups, liquids in glass ounce-sized containers, and injections in glass syringes—precariously lined up on cafeteria-sized aluminum trays and passing them to forty patients, on time, which was a tremendous feat of organization for a student nurse's first experience.

Had I been complimented on that? I don't remember. What I do remember is the silly little incident of the IV pole.

On another day I stifled gags as I inhaled whiffs of mouthwash and bedpans while I waited for another instructor, a woman who bounced side to side as she stood by the nurses' station, to give me my bath assignment. Ever moving, she punctuated her sentences with a giggle and a slap on her thigh. Pointing at me, she said. "Miss Hoitenga, I have assigned you Mr. Jacobs, age thirty-five, in 214 Bed 2—that's in the corner of the five-bed ward. He's cracked his fifth cervical vertebra, so he's flat on his back with his neck in Crutchfield Tongs. You must remember not to roll the head of the bed up. And, because he's immobile, he will be a complete bath."

In the nursing arts lab, we had learned different types of bath procedures: partial and complete. Partial, I knew, we did back and legs; the patient did the rest, including the genital area. Complete—I scanned my mind for the procedure, at least a full page in my procedure book—we did it all. Taking a breath, I stared her down as if this were an everyday happening.

I had never seen a man naked before. In the lab we had practiced baths on manikins, female ones, with no attachments. I methodically got my basin of warm water from the small bathroom next to Bed 1, hand-tested it for temperature, then crowded behind the corner curtain of Bed 2.

"Mr. Jacobs, my name is Miss Hoitenga. I am your student nurse for today, and I'll be giving you your bath." I spoke to his chin because the tongs on either side of his head limited his vision to the ceiling.

Before he could say anything, I began perfectly performing every memorized step of my procedure book version of the complete bath. "Would you like soap on your face?"

He said "yes" to the ceiling. He had tanned skin and dark eyelashes, reminding me of my sixth-grade crush, Joe, who now sat on my dorm bed in the stuffed-dog form of Joe-Marv. I felt a flutter in my throat. I had never taken care of a man this young before.

I concentrated on the procedure: start with the face. If the patient can't wash his own, ask if he wants soap. I fashioned the washcloth into the pre-scribed mitt by folding it in thirds over my shaking right fingers—leaving my thumb free—and tucking the flap under the fold on my palm. It had been dif-ficult enough learning how to make the mitt, but now, as I undid and remade the thumbless mitten each time to rinse it out, my fingers stumbled awkwardly over themselves.

Giving a bath should take about twenty minutes. Not that one. About one hour, limited conversation, and several basins of water later, I finished all but Mr. Jacob's personal bath. I wished desperately he was a partial bath, so I could leave. But no luck. I made the final trip to the bathroom in the corner of the ward for fresh water.

When I returned, I said, "Mr. Jacobs, I'm going to finish your bath now." Still looking at the ceiling, he mumbled "okay." I pulled back the sheet and uncov-ered his genitalia, obviously not expecting my virgin hands. He said nothing more, a thirty-five-year-old man held captive by an eighteen-year-old co-ed.

I focused on the procedure: lather the soap, fold the mitt, wash. My palm filled with his wobbling flaccid—I couldn't even think the word. I stroked down-ward. Hair. I had no idea hair grew on the scrotum. Had there been a picture in my textbook I'd repressed? I tried to lather its circumference, but it, too, bobbled left and right, testes falling in and out of my mitt. Settling for semi-success, I shook out the cloth in the basin of water to rinse out the soap, and then I returned my mitted hand to rinse off the soap.

I rinsed, but the lather stayed.

Remaining silent, Mr. Jacobs scanned the ceiling tiles. His tanned chin seemed to get darker. His arms lay still at his sides. I wished I could hand him the rag, but I was too befuddled to speak.

The procedure book hadn't said anything about a soap-caked scrotum. I didn't think I should touch this thing with my free bare hand, so I tried to hold everything steady with my right hand constrained in the mitt. It was like juggling tennis balls from pinkie to thumb, hoping they wouldn't drop down to the bed. But they did. After them I went, gently nudging the underside to complete des-oaping once and for all. I was engrossed in the soapy scrotal hair when my peripheral vision caught sight of a gigantic leaning tower. All expression flew from my face as I felt my fingers stiffen.

My mother's Kotex-birds-and-bees lecture to me at age eleven hadn't prepared me for fleshy uprisings. For an eternal second, the tower and I stood together—in awed silence. I grabbed a towel, jiggled Mr. Jacob's genitals dry, flipped the bath blanket over him, yanked the curtain open a crack, and fled with soapy water sloshing side-to-side in my basin.

Charging the door to the hallway, I bumped into the orderly, dark-haired and swarthy. He grabbed the doorframe for balance and said, "Is Mr. Jacobs ready for his personal bath?"

What on earth, I thought. I stared at him and blurted, "I did it."

Vincent grinned. "You're kidding; I always do all the personal baths of the men on this floor. Didn't the instructor tell you?"

I didn't dare tell my instructor. I was sure she'd nail me for not knowing my procedure. And I couldn't risk her reading any animosity on my face if she should hint at indiscretion on my part. Even though I pictured that instructor, with her sense of humor, slapping her thigh with the news, I fled to the basement cafeteria to tell a few classmates over lunch. "Guess what happened to me this morning!" Howls of laughter skipped across the lunch tables.

But the final laugh was on me when I got back to my dorm room and reviewed the procedure for a male complete bath. I hadn't recalled step twenty-one, "If he requires assistance, obtain an orderly." In my mind, I gave myself credit for completing the other twenty-three steps correctly.

On another unit, a dark-haired, serious instructor approached me in the hallway after I'd completed my morning assignment: "I've got good news, Miss Hoitenga. Your patient's doctor was just in and ordered a soapsuds enema. I think you still need the experience, right?"

As students, we carried a personal *Clinical Experience Manual* to each ward so the instructor could check what procedures we still needed to demonstrate. After we'd completed the procedure under her supervision, she would sign off in a column labeled "Satisfactory Performance."

I reviewed the half-page of the procedure in my mind and got the supplies from the utility room: a 1000cc graduated pitcher (a quart-sized metal can looking like a giant measuring cup), a plastic rectal tube, and a metal funnel. In the pitcher, I mixed up 30cc of soapsuds concentrate with 1000cc of warm water, hand testing it to be sure it was between 105-110 degrees. After squeezing a dab of lubricant on a paper towel, I headed, with all my supplies on a tray, instructor alongside, to the patient's room.

"You'll have to turn on your left side, Mrs. Barlow." As I surveyed her buttocks, I was relieved not to have to deal with a male body. My instructor stood on my right, watching every move. After attaching one end of the enema tube to the funnel and lubricating the other end, I lifted the upper buttock to see where I was going and inserted the tube exactly four inches into the rectum.

"Take deep breaths now, slowly, in and out," I said. With my left hand, I held the funnel at the level of my chest, about one foot above the rectum, according to procedure. With my right hand, I slowly started to pour the warm soapsuds into the funnel, slanted sideways so air could escape. I was proud of myself, following each step in the procedure book just as I'd practiced, without water, on our Sally Chase manikin in the nursing arts lab.

Suddenly, the tube slipped out of the rectum. Sudsy bubbles shot on the patient, on the bed, on the floor, on me, on the instructor. What was wrong?

Dumbfounded, I kept pouring.

My procedure was impeccable, but my responses not yet automatic. Soapy water continued to squirt like jumping fountains. I watched, mesmerized, as if I were seeing the Lake Michigan water show at Grand Haven. Lucky for me and the patient, my instructor, a pained expression on her face, pinched the tubing in half.

The show was over. I started to laugh, but stopped quickly with the reprimand: "You should've held on to the tube, Miss Hoitenga." No smile. Couldn't she see that the unexpected shower was funny? It hadn't hurt anyone.

How could I have held on, I yelled silently, *when I had to use one hand to hold the funnel and the other hand to pour from the can?* Where was I supposed to get another hand? Much later, I learned to avoid enema fountains by standing on one leg and securing the tubing between my raised knee and the mattress.

But that day I squelched any retort. Someday, when my attitude no longer mattered, I told myself, I'd get back at these instructors somehow.

Toward the end of my junior year, I got to my operating room rotation. With thoughts of Cherry Ames, surgical nurse, I'd fantasized about that day. To be away for awhile from passing meds, changing dressings, and starting IVs. To be safe from making mistakes that might harm or kill a patient. To have the instructor out of sight most of the time.

On my first day, the instructor, a drill sergeant in green scrubs, assigned me to assist a scrub nurse in a major surgery. No simple hernia, tonsils, or appendix, but a surgery that would take hours and involve an operating room full of assistants.

I shivered in the chilly hallway as I stared at my name on the assignment sheet. I reminded myself there was no reason to be scared: I would be working next to a nurse and she would be helping me. Even so, I felt a bit shaky.

The instructor had drilled us on sterile technique. We repeatedly practiced washing our hands, gowning with the help of a circulating nurse, and putting on our gloves without contaminating them. Now I needed to do these things for real. Quaking with goose bumps, I entered the scrub room—a small room outside the operating room. Disinfectant odors mixed dizzily with my scrambled egg breakfast I'd eaten in the cafeteria.

Following the multi-stepped procedure firmly outlined in my mind, I tucked my pixie-cut hair into a cotton skullcap and tied it at the nape of my neck. I placed a gauze mask over my nose, draped the upper strings over my ears, and tied them at the back of my head. Then I flattened the lower strings along my cheeks and tied them also at the nape of my neck.

As I took breaths, the gauze mask filled with moisture. My face got hot, and I felt as if I would suffocate. I stuck out my tongue to push the mask off my lips and open up an air pocket below my nose to breathe.

With my right knee, I felt for the faucet under the sink. Nudging it carefully to get the right stream of water and using an oblong brush and pHisoHex, I scrubbed under my nails and each area of my hands and forearms thirty times. Then, to keep clean, I hugged my elbows to my waist and raised my hands, palms up, shoulder height. I could feel my arm muscles quiver in anticipation.

I drip-dried as I backed through the door into the operating room. The circulating nurse helped me put on a sterile gown, and, following the proper procedure, I slipped on the sterile gloves she'd laid out for me. Clasping my hands above my waist, I stood ready, the picture of perfect sterile technique.

Staff flitted around like ghosts. Noises hissed from behind the drape where the anesthesiologist monitored the sleeping patient. I breathed in an unfamiliar odor—was it ether? When I breathed out, it felt as if its heavy sweetness mixed with the moisture under my mask to form a paste on my cheeks.

Ghostly silence crowded the room. Suddenly, a circulating nurse shouted across the room to me. "He's on his way. You glove him."

A world-famous surgeon. Jitters skipped through my body. Wrapped in green with only my eyes showing, I looked like a grasshopper in my starchy-smelling scrubs but felt very important—my debut as a surgical nurse imminent. An event to call home about that night.

I rechecked the layout of the surgeon's gloves on the sterile table and reran the gloving procedure through my mind. The steps were clear. I was all set. In those days, I instinctively knew I was not supposed to upset a doctor in any way. Doctors were our bread and butter—if they didn't admit their patients to our hospital, nurses wouldn't have patients. And without patients, nurses wouldn't have jobs. And without jobs, nurses wouldn't have paychecks—nurses' salaries were lumped in with the room rates. So we took what now qualifies as verbal harassment. And we jumped from our chairs in the nurses' station to give doctors a seat when they marched in. And we also stood aside as they got on and off elevators before us.

I was ready to jump for this surgeon.

Turning my head to watch for his arrival, I stared at the swinging door. All breathing stopped when he swooped into the room. All eyes watched him parade toward me. All eyes watched me as I cuffed a glove carefully over my fingers, positioned my hands above my waist, and waited for the dive of his hand.

Looking at my hands, he plunged his hand into the glove and, abruptly, flipped his hand up in front of his face. Empty rubber fingers flopped in the air. None of his fingers had found the right places.

His eyes swept the room.

I realized, instantly, I'd gloved his right hand with a left glove. His icy stare hit me like an avalanche. Before I could recover, he shouted at the interns and residents and nurses standing on the other side of the anesthetized patient: "Damn this student. Didn't anybody teach her how to put on gloves?"

"Her." That was me. Feeling myself go pale, I knew I had to try again. Just that fast, the circulating nurse had flipped open another package of gloves on the sterile table. Mortified and nearly numb with fright, I quickly picked up another glove and slowly repeated the procedure, correctly the second time.

I did not tell my instructor. In her military manner, I could hear her clipped phrases about not paying attention. Maybe she'd laugh, but I couldn't take the chance. So the only comfort I got was an eyebrow twitch above her mask from the scrub nurse, as if to say, "Get used to it."

That evening, June 19, 1961, I wrote in my diary: "My first day of scrubbing in surgery—quite nervous. Glove wrong."

I did not call home. There was nothing good to report about my failed debut.

Pranks are not nursing procedures, exactly. But they are things I learned, as a newcomer to living away from home. Pranks, like nursing procedures, involved a lot of steps to execute and provided an optimal distraction from my supposed attitude problem on the ward.

Early on, coming back to my room from supper, I was surprised to find a lonely Kotex pad lying on the bare springs of my bed. A note sprawled on the springs read: "Sorry. I washed your mattress and it shrunk." I decided to first look in the closet. Since the closet wasn't deep, I knew to open the door carefully. Sure enough, my mattress, sheets hanging askew—no contour sheets in those days—smashed my hanging clothes and was ready to spring forward and knock me over. Being the lucky recipient of that prank taught me how it was done, so I could do it proficiently to others and, from the pranks that followed, to learn how I could reciprocate.

Some pranks could only take place at night. Once, in a midnight stupor, sitting on the toilet in the communal bathroom, I felt warm liquid streaming down my legs. Only to discover plastic wrap under the seat, stretched over the top rim of the toilet bowl. And to find no one to blame at that hour except the winking face in the moon. And to have to mop up the floor and to take a shower in the lineup of shower stalls to feel clean enough to go back to bed.

The most creative surprise was some sort of initiation: a person behind me tied a cloth over my eyes behind my head, led me a few feet across a room— maybe the nursing arts lab—and said, "Get down on your hands and knees, put your right hand into this bowl, and identify what you feel." Gingerly dropping my hand inch by inch, I ran into a cold liquid. "Further down," the female voice said. I felt a cool china rim under my armpit. My hand hit the bottom of the bowl and bumped into a slimy semi-soft curved cylinder. A banana.

Banana splits have never tasted the same.

Bloody pranks worked well, too. It was great fun to kidnap Sally Chase, the practice manikin, from the nursing arts lab in the dorm's basement. We'd carry her over our backs, her legs and arms dangling, up the stairwell to the second or third floor, and slide her under a classmate's bed while she was gone to supper. Then we'd pull one leg out from under the bed and drip ketchup on it in a jagged line. We'd wait in the next room with the door cracked open. We'd hear a scream over the transom. Then shouts down the hallway, "Okay, who did it? Who did it?" We—it took two to get Sally up and down in the fastest fashion to lessen our chances of getting caught—had to quickly confess and hoist Sally back down to her bed in the lab before she was missed.

The best prank...or the worst...we carried out one day when probies moved in. A few of us went into their second-floor rooms before they arrived. Three boards supported the naked black-and-white-striped mattresses on the bed frame, one at each end, one in the middle. We removed the end boards and put them in the closet so they could easily be found. Then, balancing the mattress on the center board, we slanted it slightly sideways so opposite sides of the top and bottom would rest on the edges of the bed frame, making the mattress look sturdy. We retreated to our upper floors and waited. When we heard parents unloading cars at the basement level, we stationed ourselves on the landing of the upper stairwell. Since the only elevator was quickly tied up, we could see the tops of heads and a collection of boxes, stuffed animals, and hanging clothes making their way up the stairs. Soon we heard an array of thudding noises and imagined an unsuspecting mother, arms full, collapsing on the foot end of a bed. In our minds we saw the bed become a teeter-totter as her head would *almost* clunk on the far side of the bed frame and her legs would come to rest on the near side, pointing to the ceiling. Then we heard a man's voice yelling, "Good heavens. Someone could get killed just moving in here." Heavy footsteps followed, flying down the lower stairwell. Our stifled giggles stopped instantly when we suspected we were being reported.

Since the nursing director couldn't know who was responsible, she summoned the whole slew of us upperclassmen to the dorm's living room on the first floor. Surrounded by the formal brocade furniture supplied by the women's guild, we sat cross-legged on the floor waiting for her arrival. It was the same place we'd sat a few months before watching the launching of the first manned Mercury mission on a small-screened TV console. That had been more fun.

The director arrived in her full white starched splendor, the picture of professionalism, a slender woman with perfectly coiffed auburn hair and perfectly outlined red lips. "Something very upsetting has happened. It could have been catastrophic. A parent could have been dangerously injured…."

I pictured a mother jackknifed on the downed mattresses, suppressed a grin, and wondered why the parents didn't look in the closet, see the humor, and fix the problem without reporting us. But I had no appreciation at the time of how dangerous our prank was. Caught up in group fun, I don't suppose any of us thought of people getting hurt. After the nursing director's scolding, we scurried like naughty mice from the room, scampered single file up the stairway to the snack bar, closed the door, and burped out our suppressed giggles.

That prank was not an event I'd call home about. My folks would not be pleased with this fun-gone-overboard behavior. It was a long while before I got over my fear of being found out. And before I felt properly sorry.

But I was never sorry for any of the other pranks. Our laughter was enormously cathartic.

By our senior year, we were comfortable seeing autopsies and would stop in on our way to supper to see if there was anything exciting. Ward 20, the morgue, was across from the cafeteria so it was easy to run in to check. One afternoon, the body of a young man lay naked on the table, his face covered with scalp skin pulled forward like a mask. A clot of blood, resembling a tablespoon of black cherry Jell-O, nestled into the cream-colored, macaroni-like brain tissue. The pathologist told us this was a teenager who died in a motorbike accident. He pointed to the clot: "This is a subdural hematoma."

I crossed my arms tightly to protect myself from the assaulting news. My first brain, my first hematoma, my first young death. From a motorbike accident. The room swirled as I breathed in the formaldehyde odor, shivered in the stark cold, and stared at the body lying on the shiny, narrow chrome table. Taking several deep breaths, I focused on the pathologist performing his exam and tape-recording his findings.

Back at the dorm after supper, I called home to tell my folks. "Hello." My mother sounded business-like.

"Hi, Mother." My voice broke as I inhaled the smell of formaldehyde still clinging to my starched uniform.

"Lois, I'm glad you called." Her matter-of-fact tone told me she had something to tell me. "Your second cousin, David Vermeer, was in an awful motorbike accident today. His friend was killed."

I stiffened. I didn't know the patient's name from the autopsy and, of course, hadn't seen his face. But how many motorbike accidents could happen in one day? Even though I didn't know David, and only faintly remembered his parents, my pork chop and applesauce supper jumped toward my throat.

My mother rambled on about the accident. "But David got broken bones and was admitted to your hospital. Would you stop in to see him?"

I dashed through the archway over to the hospital and checked in at the front desk to find out his room number. Room 201, a private room, darkened at that twilight hour, across from the nurses' station. I stopped in the doorway. A strange teenager lay in the shadows of the hall light. What could I say to this young driver of a motorbike whose friend had been killed? Since I didn't know him, I felt detached, not like a distant relative. I made small talk about his legs suspended in complicated ropes of traction and how long he'd be hanging up like that.

I left, feeling I had a long way to go before I could ever be able to be a good nurse. I now knew how to do procedures, dozens of them, but didn't know how to talk to patients in their worst time of need. Shouldn't I have learned somewhere along the way how to respond appropriately?

But maybe I had been taught something and my attitude stuff had gotten in the way. I surely wasn't going to confide in any instructor now about feeling inadequate.

On Easter of my senior year, I worked a day shift, 7:00 to 3:30, in the emergency room. I scowled through the day. I'd rather have been home hearing my dad's sermon and eating my mother's ham and apple pie on the holiday. At last three o'clock rolled around. Several of us students stood leaning on the nurses' station, passing time. It had been a slow day. Not many patients. Wanting to break the monotony, I quipped, "The only thing that could happen now is someone coming in who choked on Easter dinner."

A siren screamed up the driveway. The double doors opened. Ambulance attendants pushed in a stretcher, head first. I saw an old man's head—lifeless and blue. DOA: dead on arrival. An elderly woman, dressed in Easter egg pink, followed. "Help him, please! He choked…." She hobbled behind the stretcher, mopping her eyes, wailing, "Please, help him."

My joke had caused this man's death—I was sure.

I felt myself turn white. I clutched the counter of the nurses' station. As the room spun around me, I grabbed shallow breaths and forced swallows to fight down nausea.

While the ER staff took care of the patient, I sat with his wife, Mrs. Hattie Wellington. She gripped my hand and begged for assurance that the staff would save him. I couldn't think of what to say, so I placed my hand over hers. After a long while, a nurse came. Her eyes spoke "death." Mrs. Wellington's voice erupted into screams.

There was a full-page procedure we'd learned for care of the dead, but we'd not learned how to care for their family members. I sat silently while the nurse invited Mrs. Wellington to go with her to see her husband. I stayed behind, frozen in my chair. I don't remember telling anyone about my careless quip concerning death. I don't remember an instructor even being with us that day. It was perhaps a typical thing to say for a twenty-year-old, but not appropriate for a person to say who'd been entrusted with the serious matters of life and death. The statement would not have helped any evaluation of my attitude.

At 3:30 we were able to go off duty on time. The patient rode on a cart to the morgue. Mrs. Wellington, draped in damp pink on her children's arms, shuffled to their car in the parking lot. We ambled in silence to early supper in the cafeteria. The usual whiff of formaldehyde from the morgue across the hall permeated our Easter dinner of baked ham, sweet potatoes, and peas and preserved the memory forever.

A few weeks after that Easter, I found an official-looking note in my student mailbox. My eyes widened. I'd been lucky; I hadn't had any scary notes since my invitation to an appointment with the director informing me of my demotion and since I'd been given a warning about my apron desecration. I took the folded paper and slipped it behind the bib of my uniform apron so I could wait to read it until I got to my room. Once there, I unbuttoned the back waist of my apron, shimmied my arms out of the bib, let the apron slip to the floor, flopped on my bed in my pin-striped dress, and slowly unfolded the note. What could it possibly say now? It was not even four months to graduation. Surely, I couldn't be expelled at this late date.

I blinked as I read the note a second time: "Miss Hoitenga, I am very happy to be able to tell you that the faculty has selected you to assist us this summer in the clinical supervision of the freshman students. We will contact you later for orientation to your duties." The note was dated May 24, 1962, and signed by the assistant director with the dates of the assignment written in the bottom left hand corner: "July 2 to August 6."

Me, the student with the attitude problem! By a mysterious miracle, my attempts at sprucing up my attitude had apparently worked. There must have been encouraging clues from my instructors, but my mind, full of worry about whether my attitude was going to pass inspection, had simply not heard them. And now, that same "attitude problem" me had been chosen to be an instructor for the probies!

I called my folks. Dad answered. I told him the news, then added, "Thanks, Dad, for making me stay." I jokingly reminded him of all the times I had called home wanting to quit. Especially that first smelly summer on Men's Ward.

I could hear tears in his voice as he cleared his throat. "Yes, yes. My, my. Congratulations! I'll hand the phone to Mother."

"Hello, now what?" Mother asked. I don't think she dared hope for good news.

"Mother, I may be a teacher yet. I've been selected to be a student instructor this summer." As she asked what that involved, I could feel her smile.

Cherry Ames, teacher. I was on my way. I'd help students when they messed up. I'd help them have fun learning to become a nurse. I might even teach them about dorm pranks—safe ones, that is. And if they started having attitude problems, I'd do my best to walk with them through the bad times. After all, I'd had experience.

Three

SHIFT WORK

should have known in nurses' training when I needed to pray to start the day that this need would not disappear after graduation.

At Blodgett, new graduates got the night shift. There was a saying that went like this: "You won't get days unless someone retires or dies." It was a hierarchy. The new grad worked herself down the clock from nights to PMs to days. As senior students, we'd plotted in our minds how to incapacitate a few of the older day-shift RNs. We usually wouldn't kill them outright. A small accident would do, one that would break a leg and take months to heal. Enough time to hasten our jump down the clock.

My night shifts as a new grad started, unofficially, the day Marv and I got married. My dad had married us at two in the afternoon on September 8, 1962, the day after my graduation, in my church in Cutlerville, a block down 68th Street from Pine Rest and my first patients, Greta and Tryntje. A memorable day for me, until that evening in Ludington, about a hundred miles north, in a musty log cabin. After I'd taken a picture, black and white, of our newly ringed hands and my pink roses corsage on the white chenille spread, Marv had a sudden bout of vomiting. Then he passed out on the bed. While he snored, I lovingly turned off the overhead light so I wouldn't bother my brand-new husband and camped out in the bathroom to read, sandwiched between the tub and the toilet on a cold tiled floor. I suppose I read tourist magazines; I surely would not have brought along any novels, and I tiptoed back hourly to check his pulse and breathing.

I didn't know then he could sleep through fireworks. And I didn't know that others, like him, who had stayed at one of his sisters' the night before the wedding, were throwing up. They never did track the cause. And I guess by that time I was used to people being sick, because I don't remember being bothered by my wedding night not turning out as I'd hoped.

Marv and I settled into a seventy-five-dollar-a-month, second-floor apartment of an old frame house at 447 Fuller in Grand Rapids, a few miles from Blodgett and a few blocks from Calvin. Marv was a senior that fall and had a part-time job building garages. The Tuesday after our wedding I stood up in my roommate Kate's wedding. The next week I started my official night duty on my favorite floor, Hall Two West. The same floor where I'd given my first male bath. The same floor with the jolly instructor who'd slapped her thigh in delight. The same floor where I'd visited my second cousin who had been in the accident that killed his friend. Medical-surgical. Twenty-seven beds. A range of room sizes (private to a five-bed ward) meeting at a corner nurses' station. I liked the variety of patients: those with diabetes, cataract extractions, thyroidectomies, radical mastectomies, fractured bones pinned and in traction, and more. I liked the challenge of change. I liked action.

I also went back to Calvin, taking one course at a time that would apply someday toward a bachelor's degree. Nurses' training had overdosed my mind in the sciences; I still wanted the liberal arts courses I hadn't had because my folks had said no to my going to a four-year degree program.

Life was supposed to be great. But, as newlyweds, Marv and I suffered through a love-starved schedule of musical beds—me in, him out; him in, me out. We saw each other awake for only a few minutes each evening, and on the every third weekend I had off. I envied a group of my classmates who had moved into a house together after graduation. They worked nights, too, and, afterward, went home and unloaded their stories on each other, with much hilarity, over breakfast. When they invited me, I loved the laughter. After breakfast, I went to our empty apartment, only a few blocks away, and missed the camaraderie.

One morning I drove home from work and parked by the garage in the back of the house. The upstairs was dark. Marv had either already left for work or for an eight o'clock class. Sometimes I could catch him home for five minutes, but not that day. I unlocked the back door and began climbing the dark, stuffy stairway. Stumbling on the torn rubber matting on the third step, I fell to my knees. Tears came. I pushed myself up and trudged, step by step, the rest of the way, feeling very sorry for myself. What kind of life was this for a new bride? There was no way out. I was doomed to night duty, and Marv's schedule was days.

As much as I hated leaving for work at 10:30 p.m., once I got there I was fine. There was something about the grandeur of the stairwell to Hall Two. Worn granite steps, sky-high ceilings, smells of the five-story, red-brick, 1916 building. The hall lights on West Two were dimmed at this hour of the night. Within minutes I was behind the steel desk in the supervisor's office getting report from the weary PM nurse who had been in charge of both West and East ends of the floor—fifty-five patients.

I listened to report for about twenty to thirty minutes. I asked questions. I clarified things I didn't understand. My mind raced, juggling all the information. My list of things to check or do grew and grew. Minutes before, my head had been empty and filled with nighttime darkness; now fact upon fact saturated my brain. I felt jolted into fluorescent light awareness.

After report, I chitchatted a bit with the PM nurse. Not long, though. We both felt rushed, she to cross off the last tasks on her list—maybe starting an IV for one of her two meds nurses, noting a doctor's order on a late admission, ensuring no visitors were still on the floor—and me to start making rounds to see each of my twenty-seven patients.

I started out of the nurses' station with my clipboard scribbled full—names, diagnoses, treatments. As I entered each room, I shone my flashlight over each person's chest, watching for even and regular up and down movement. If the patient was awake, I introduced myself. "Hi, Mrs. Jones, my name is Mrs. Roelofs." As nurses, we still used our last names then.

Shining my flashlight on my clipboard to refresh my memory, I'd say, "I'm the night nurse on this floor. I'm here to check your…" Say it was her IV, catheter, and dressing. I whispered and checked at the same time. I checked her arm. "Your IV is running well. There's no sign of redness or swelling on your arm. No infection." I lifted the linens to check her dressing. "Your dressing is dry. That means there's no drainage we can see." I followed the tubing of her catheter down to the drainage bag hanging on the frame of the bed. "We want to make sure you're getting enough fluids. Your urine is a little dark yet. If you're awake during the night, sip this water here." I scooted the bedside table within her reach. "One last thing. Let me help you cough while I'm here. We don't want you to get pneumonia."

It was important to move quickly, to fly from bed to bed. There were meds to give at midnight and blood pressures to take on the post-ops, and insulins to give the newly diagnosed diabetics on a 12-6-12-6 feeding routine. Unless I was charting or ordering medication refills or checking twenty-four-hour doctors' orders for accuracy against the Kardex (a flip-open file of patient information), I rarely sat again until giving report to the day shift at seven.

Once my rounds were completed, I felt better, my body de-escalated from ultra-tense to semi-tense. Even so, I never completely relaxed, staying in a state of hyper-vigilance. I'd learned my lesson well; as a senior student, I was sent once from one floor to another during report, to a floor with which I was unfamiliar, to work alone with an aide. I missed a room on my midnight rounds, found it on three o'clock rounds, and the fear that overtook me until I was certain the four patients in that room were not face down on the floor, not hemorrhaging, and not dead still makes me shiver today.

After a year of nights, I got "promoted" to PMs. I'd had enough experience to assume charge nurse of both the West and East nurses' stations. I was thrilled to be off nights, but Marv was picking up extra classes and had the same schedule, so our game of musical beds continued. We could count on seeing each other awake on Sunday mornings and on the every third weekend I had off.

After a year of PMs, my head nurse called me into the office and told me the supervisor was leaving and she was taking the job. In the next breath, she offered me her head nurse position on our ward, Two West. This meant days—at last. Only two years to get there and no one had to die or break a leg for the miracle to happen. I skipped home to tell Marv.

I thought I would be happy, content, and well adjusted at last. But no luck. I had never been able to fall asleep after working. I'd relive the shift, making sure I didn't forget anything—a prep for an x-ray, the signed permit for surgery, a med ordered to be given at an odd time.

No matter how hard I prayed, sleep came only when my shift was finished a second time.

On the day shift, I thought I would have the whole evening to rework my day in my head, so I should be able to drift off to sleep. But, I invented a new worry: whether I'd wake up to my alarm. Perfecting this worry, I woke up every day without the alarm, way too early. I would not dare to doze to catch another dream before the alarm went off, because my worry center knew any sleep would turn into a nightmare about being late for work. A nightmare of rushing out of bed, running my support nylons while yanking them on, not having time to shower or to press my 100-percent cotton long-sleeved uniform for a second day's wear, and generally being discombobulated for the day.

Getting up at 5:30 in the morning never was easy. But, as usual, once I got to the hospital, I'd thrive on the excitement: patients coming and going to tests or surgery, doctors flitting in and out of the nurses' station, and me noting the doctors' orders with the help of a ward clerk. The day would go by fast. No sooner would I come back from lunch than it'd be time to make afternoon rounds and get ready to give report to the PM shift.

One afternoon while making rounds, I dashed in to see Mr. Barnes, my last patient, in 236-1, the triple ward next to the nurses' station. He smiled when he saw me. "I'm going out for dinner tonight. Dr. Jericho is picking me up at five."

"Oh? I didn't know. He didn't tell us at the desk," I said, scanning the patient's Kardex card in the vertical file positioned on my left arm. "I'll check on it."

Back at the nurses' station, I checked the doctor's order sheet for Mr. Barnes. Hospital policy dictated that patients could leave hospital grounds only with written orders from their attending physician. Dr. Jericho was not the attending physician; he was a personal friend. And there was no written order. Had he cleared taking Mr. Barnes out with the attending physician?

I faced a potential explosion. Dr. Jericho's capacity to be short-tempered was well known to the nursing staff. We'd each had our experiences. None of us liked it, but we felt powerless to do any more than endure. And I didn't need the problem right then: I wanted to give report on time and get home on time for once. I quickly dialed his office. "Hello, Dr. Jericho, this is Mrs. Roelofs on Hall Two. Your friend, Joseph Barnes, told me you were picking him up for dinner." I swallowed hard and took a breath. "I see no written order covering this leave. I'm calling to see if you've run this by his attending, Dr. Acorn."

He barked into my eardrum. "I don't need to check anything out with anybody. Do you hear me? It's none of your business…. Who is this again? What's your name?"

"Mrs. Roelofs. Head nurse. Hall Two." I forced my voice to sound strong.

"I'm coming right over to clean your clock," Dr. Jericho yelled into the phone.

My head and heart spun wildly into one big tuft of fear that settled in my throat. I raced to a friend working on the ward at the other end of my floor. We schemed to hide me on that ward when Dr. Jericho arrived. Then we stationed lookout nurses. Minutes later I got the message. I ducked into Room 214, a five-bed room on East, and hid behind curtains drawn around a vacant bed. When Dr. Jericho arrived, my cohorts told him I was off the floor on an errand. He strode into my nurses' station across from Room 201, parked himself on my desk chair, and bellowed, "I'll wait."

When I was a student nurse a few years before, I had scrubbed to assist Dr. Jericho in surgery. He became irritated with something and kicked a metal wastebasket across the room. Anesthesia saved the patient from being startled off the operating table. However, my nerves, as a novice, vibrated with the intensity of the metal clanging against steel and tile. Now my nerves were vibrating once again.

Suddenly, my friend peeked around the curtain, wearing worry on her face. "He won't leave until he sees you. He's camped out. Slicked back hair, black suit, green paisley tie, and all. You better come."

I returned to the utility room on my ward with its steel cabinets, stowed commodes and IV poles, soaking instruments and thermometers, and corner hopper—a large square toilet-like bowl for rinsing bedpans. Standing in the doorway to the adjacent nurses' station, I said as confidently as possible, "Dr. Jericho, I'm back. I understand you want to see me?"

Dr. Jericho launched to a standing position. "You bet I do. Who do you think you are to question what I'm doing? To tell me I need a doctor's order to take my friend out for dinner?" His words torpedoed through the nurses' station and up the ramp to pediatrics.

He stomped toward me. I backed away, inch by inch, until I was flush with the hopper. One more step and I'd plop into hopper water. I was trapped. Only the smothering smells of disinfectant separated us. "It's my responsibility to see that hospital policy is followed, sir," I said. My breath stopped momentarily.

"Who are you to tell me what hospital policy says? You, young lady, are never to question me again. Do you understand?"

His words slapped my face like sleet on a winter walk. I could have punched him—he was close enough—but I thought better of it. "Yes, sir." I held back a salute that he seemed to demand. He turned, clicked his heels, and marched out, as if on a military drill.

My meds nurse, LPN, and aides crowded into the small nurses' station. "What happened? What'd he say? I've never seen him so mad. At least not this week."

"Oh, the usual Dr. Jericho stuff. Nothing new." I said, trying to sound nonchalant with a heart rate of over a hundred. Reaching for the desk phone, I glanced at a list of phone numbers and dialed Mr. Barnes' attending physician. He gave me the order. Why hadn't I called him in the first place?

I determined never to let a doctor's behavior intimidate me again.

"Roly!" As I heard my nickname called, I turned to see Dr. Salmon, another surgeon, coming out of Room 202 next to the nurses' station. "Roly, when you have time, would you irrigate my patient's Levine tube? Al Merrill. Bed three.

Something must be stuck in his gut because it's not draining as easily as I'd like to see, and I have an emergency in ER."

"Are you sure? You've written a strict 'Do not irrigate' order." I flipped open the Kardex to make sure. "And you've noted that you don't want the nurses touching that tube."

"Yeah, I know. I'm a fanatic about guarding my delicate internal sutures. But I know you'll do it safely." And off he went, dressed in green scrubs and skullcap, up the ramp through pediatrics to the elevator down to ER.

The wall clock said 2:30 p.m. Seven minutes left until I needed to give report. Just enough time. I returned to the utility room to get a sterile irrigation tray. Balancing the cloth-wrapped tray on my hands, I strode happily down the hall into Room 202.

Four

ROTTEN POTATOES

*H*oney, I think we better move to Minneapolis. Shell Personnel called today and said they could find me a job. Even though I'm I-A."

It was the fall of 1965, the height of the Vietnam War, and the placement company had not been able to find Marv a job in Grand Rapids after he'd graduated in May. He was third on his home county's list in Minnesota for being called and was passing time working in the freezer of a meat packing plant. A few weeks before, he'd gone to an interview in Chicago and had been offered a job as a juvenile court probation officer. The prospect of living in Chicago excited us. When we'd traveled through the city to visit his folks over the years, Marv always commented, "This is the heartbeat of the nation. I can actually feel a beat-beat-beat." But then he turned the job down. "We can't live on that salary, honey." Fifty-five hundred. So we packed a twenty-foot U-Haul box truck, pulled our 1960 Beetle behind it, and moved to Minneapolis.

Wanting experience in a smaller hospital, I chose one within walking distance from our one-bedroom garden apartment. It was a sixty-seven-bed hospital where I had to rotate all three shifts in one week. I worked 11-7 on Sunday and Monday, 3-11 on Wednesday and Thursday, and a double-back to 7-3 on Friday. My body didn't adjust; it never knew whether it was supposed to sleep or be awake. I was tired all the time.

My fluffy-white-haired head nurse wore spotless square-heeled shoes and a floral hanky fanned in the breast pocket of her starched uniform dress. She looked like an advertisement for Griffin shoe polish and Niagara starch. When I looked at her, I'd be tempted to shove my scuffed flat-soled shoes in her face and twirl the drawstrings at the waist of my wash-and-wear uniform up in the air.

When I'd worked there a week, I asked her if I could be assigned to the four-bed intensive care ward that was part of our floor. "No," she said, fingering her rhinestone-studded pen. "You are too young and haven't had enough experience yet."

I wanted to strangle her. This hospital was archaic compared to Blodgett. During nurses' training, I had worked in a brand-new intensive care unit, not a converted ward like this one, taking care of patients with burns, tracheotomies, and multiple fractures. As a graduate, I'd run wards with patients sicker than she might have ever seen.

One morning she assigned me to a prominent woman in town, a socialite, who was "up and about" and in for tests. "Give her a complete bath," she said. "She expects it."

I had not become a nurse to pamper the wealthy. I had learned that nursing is about helping patients help themselves. I resigned. I had worked there only five weeks.

No job materialized for Marv. Too risky for hire with a draft status of I-A. He took a grad course in statistics at the University of Michigan, sprayed dandelions, and attempted to sell encyclopedias, while I took a job as a Kelly Girl.

This wasn't the lifestyle we'd hoped for.

"What can you do?" the Kelly Girl receptionist said when I told her I was a nurse. She decided the only skills I had that she could use were an ability to read and to alphabetize. "We'll start you with proofreading the Yellow Pages," she said. "When that job finishes, I'll put you into filing." It took sixty endless minutes of reading the Yellow Pages to pay for each day's lunch at Dayton's cafeteria. I still appreciate a Yellow Page ad neatly encased in a black-outlined square with no spelling errors.

Because we were certain Marv would soon be drafted, we decided that he, as a college grad, should enlist in the Army as a second lieutenant. The recruiter promised that if I enlisted, we'd stay together. As a nurse, I'd be a first lieutenant. *Ha, ha*, we thought. Marv would have to salute me! We were told we'd both be assigned in Denver, me to Fitzsimmons Hospital.

We never finished the paperwork.

"We're moving to Chicago," Marv announced on the phone. He had driven back to check out the probation officer position at Cook County's Juvenile Court he'd turned down less than a year earlier because it didn't pay enough. The morning before, when he was leaving for Chicago, he'd come into the bedroom to kiss me good-bye. I had just recorded my temperature on a grid in an old Calvin bluebook.

"Honey, my temp is up almost a whole degree."

His departure was delayed. We had been trying to get pregnant for over two years, and the promise of this temp spike could not be passed up.

The pay the Court was offering him now was millionaire pay next to my proofreading the Yellow Pages and his spraying dandelions. "We'll manage to live on it," Marv said. "I'll call Aunt Maggie to find us a place to live."

We borrowed four hundred dollars from my sister Esther, rented a U-Haul again, towed the Beetle, and moved immediately. At her invitation, we settled into Marv's aunt's basement in Cicero, a western suburb. Before his job started, Marv drove a truck on his cousin's garbage route, 2:00 a.m. to noon, in the Water Street Market. When he got home, he dropped his dirty clothes next to the washer in the basement. Rotten potatoes festered on the pant legs, and the stench seeped into our one-room suite next door.

I began to vomit and did not stop for three weeks. I lost twenty-two pounds and finally got in to see a new doctor in the Loop, recommended by my former roommate Kate. She was living up north in Skokie while her husband was in grad school. On the way to our first obstetrician visit, Marv and I stopped to drop my vomit bag in a Michigan Avenue trash can. After more than two years of monthly crying parties, the news that we were expecting sent us soaring.

We had given up that Marv would ever be reclassified to III-A, the paternity deferment President Kennedy broadened on March 14, 1963, to include all men who were fathers, not just those whose induction would cause extreme hardship. The new Executive Order 11098 covered a man's child from the date of its conception. Marv was granted his III-A status on August 3, 1966.

As soon as the worst of prenatal nausea was over, I began working at West Suburban Hospital in Oak Park, Illinois. This time, I chose to work nights. I wouldn't have to worry about how I'd feel in the morning—in fact, on the few orientation days I had at the hospital, I had to leave class to throw up.

The night McCormick Place burned, a patient put his light on to ask me to come in and watch the flames on his TV. Sitting in a bedside chair, I elevated my swollen pregnant feet, jammed into tennis shoes, on a footstool. My leather Clinic shoes were home in the closet. I worked a few extra private duty shifts, earning $27 a night. Two nights' work paid for a white wicker dressing table. Our first child, Jon Hoitenga, was born in March of 1967.

I was finally the mom I'd cried to be.

Jon was six months old when Marv began to plan to go back to school for a graduate degree in social work. The Court offered a stipend of $5,000 per year with a two-day-a-week work requirement while a student and a two-year commitment afterward. I went back to work at West Sub two evenings a week to save up in anticipation of less salary.

When Jon started walking, we became antsy to leave our second-floor apartment and get a house. Marv's supervisor at the Court told him about townhouses near his in Riverdale, a south suburb of Chicago. In 1968, I quit work, Marv started grad school at Jane Addams (University of Illinois, Circle Campus), and we moved to a newly renovated, two-story, three-bedroom townhouse on Pacesetter Parkway. An end unit of four. $15,000; $500 down; FHA approved. "We can afford it, honey," Marv said. "It has a fenced yard. I want to build a sandbox and swing set for Jon."

I eagerly decorated our new living room in shades of green, starting with avocado hi-low sculptured carpeting. I was delighted to find coordinating celery, avocado, and aquamarine stripe fabric to recover a loveseat we'd lifted from someone's garbage. And to order my first custom drapes, a celery green antique satin from Penney's. The galley kitchen was yellow. The nursery, blue. I'd picked out the paint from Sears, and Marv rollered the walls while I did the trim, serenaded by old Elvis favorites: "Love Me Tender."

And soon, we were painting a second nursery pink. Kathleen Elizabeth was born in August of 1969, the summer between Marv's two years of grad school.

I still worked night shifts, but they were now at home. The only rounds I made were to the two nurseries bordering our bedroom. In the evening, Marv and I tucked the kids in together. "Now I lay me down to sleep, I pray thee, Lord, my soul to keep...."

I was married. I was a mom. I was a mom twice. And, I had nursing to fall back on if I ever needed to work.

I had everything I wanted.

Five

RUNNING AWAY

I thought I'd stay happy automatically, not working and being a full-time mom. But when Kathleen was ten months old and Jon was three, I found myself shuffling through a carpeted city of red, yellow, and blue Fisher Price blocks in the living room and walking out the front storm door. Settling into our new Opel Kadett on the driveway, I glimpsed Marv standing in the doorway, a blank expression on his face I didn't recognize. Kathleen sat on his left arm, chubby legs kicking out from her pink-striped sun suit as she waved "bye-bye to Mommy." Jon, sailor-like in navy and white shorts and T-shirt, hugged Marv's hairy legs as he pounded his "bye-bye" against the glass.

It was May of 1970. Marv was finishing his full-time graduate studies at Jane Addams. He also worked two jobs to support us. During the day, around classes and field placements, he continued his work as a probation officer, fulfilling the time required by his stipend from Cook County. Two evenings a week, he worked as a counselor for a suburban Chicago youth commission near our home. And I was leaving him, at least for the weekend, to care for our kids, the most wanted, blond-haired, blue-eyed youngsters to ever sit tandem in a double stroller on daily walks to the park—where other mothers told me what I already knew, "Your children are adorable. They look almost like twins."

I was twenty-eight years old.

I'd spent a lot of energy trying to get content. But *Sesame Street* could not compete with the books Marv was assigned to read in grad school. Since he had little time, I devoured them—*One Flew Over a Cuckoo's Nest, Black Like Me, Psychocybernetics*—and coached him over his shoulders while he typed up his papers on our old black Underwood. "I sure appreciate that you want to read all this stuff," he'd say. "I think you should be awarded the MSW along with me. You'll have earned it."

I tried taking a little course myself. When Kathleen was only a month old, I read in the local paper about an eight-session arrhythmia course at night within walking distance of our townhouse. I'd never worked in cardiac care and never wanted to, but when I mentioned it to Marv, he said, "Go for it. I'm home that night. I'd be happy to take care of the kids." The classes gave me eight nights out that re-connected the nursing circuit in my brain. And it gave me information that I've never used except to interject a sentence about QRS complexes or ST-intervals or *p* waves into conversations when I wanted to sound smart.

An oil painting class came next. Pilfering grocery money, I bought expensive Grumbacher paints, stuffed them into my boxy vinyl diaper bag, and headed off to class. But even using the best paints, I couldn't swish my still life of apples into anything more than flat circles. The second session, mid-class, I quit and came home. Seeing my face, Marv gave me a hug, shrugged, went out to the garage, and tacked my canvas of red disks, each with a curved brown stem, above his work bench.

Bowling bombed too. After joining a league as a sub, I never achieved a higher score than 118. There were no strikes and only a few spares. No one asked me to rejoin.

During naptimes, I paged feverishly through magazines—*Ladies Home Journal, McCall's, Redbook.* I read about Betty Friedan's *The Feminine Mystique* published seven years before in 1963. I searched for it on my local library's shelves, but it wasn't there. Marv checked the shelves at U of I for me, found it, and brought it home. The next afternoon I was sitting on my green striped loveseat when I read the sentence that would change my life. Something about a woman not feeling fulfilled waxing floors.

That was me. Trying to be a happy housewife, but not being successful. Friedan called it "the problem that has no name." A vague feeling of discontent. Others called the malady the "housewife syndrome." I called it restlessness. Feeling hemmed in.

At least now I knew I was not alone. Others felt like me.

I told Marv we needed a conference. He sat in his black vinyl recliner from a Fingerhut catalog while I sat opposite on the loveseat. The kids were sleeping upstairs. "I'm ready to jump out of my skin. I thought it was only me." I held up Friedan's book. "But it's not." I started to cry.

Marv handed me the handkerchief from his back pocket.

Then I poured out recent neighborhood coffee klatch conversations about pinochle clubs, diaper rash ointments, Stouffer's twice-baked potatoes. Things that didn't excite me. And never would.

Marv rearranged the newspaper on his lap. After a long silence, he said, "I wonder if you'd like to talk to a guy I met in class recently. A therapist."

A therapist! Why? Therapists were for crazy people. I wasn't crazy.

"He came to class to demonstrate techniques of Carl Rogers' client-centered therapy—mainly affirming the client's feelings. Giving the client 'unconditional positive regard.'"

Sniffling into the hanky, I felt like one big failure as a mom.

"You'd like him. I volunteered to act as a patient and, when he started talking, I immediately forgot I was a *pretend* patient."

I'd read enough of Marv's textbooks to get the gist. "It may help. I have to try something…but how will we afford it?"

"Don't worry. We'll manage."

Since I was a referral from a student, Dr. Sanderson gave me a break and charged $15 for my forty-five minutes. This older man, forty-ish seemed ancient at the time, greeted me with a warm handshake and eyes like Dennis the Menace. I liked him instantly.

He ushered me into a darkened room; two leather chairs flanked a small corner table holding the only lamp. We sat down. "So," he asked in a soft tone, "what brings you here today?"

The room felt warm and peaceful, matching his voice. There were no Legos, Lincoln Logs, or Tinker Toys on the floor here. In the dim lighting, I could only see his kindly face and a box of tissues I quickly used, one after another.

"I was raised to think I'd grow up, get married, have kids, and live happily ever after." I choked over my words. "I'm in the 'happily ever after' now, but I'm not happy."

I spent several sessions rehashing the stupidity of my neighbors who were content at home being wives and moms. Then I moved to Marv—how I hated that he was gone all the time. Finally, I got around to me, how I was mad at myself for not being the happy housewife, for feeling like the walls were caving in.

"What would make you happy?" Dr. Sanderson asked.

"Going back to school. Completing a bachelor's degree in nursing. I wanted to go for the BSN right after high school, but my folks wanted me to attend a diploma nursing program at a college associated with our church."

"So why aren't you going back to school now?"

"None of my friends at church or in my neighborhood wants to take any classes."

"I don't understand what that has to do with you," he said.

Dumb. Dumb. Dumb. I'd never thought of going back to school alone. Driving home in the rain, I clenched the steering wheel and cried. Almost scraping the side of a viaduct, I jerked the steering wheel straight. Fear pounded my forehead. How could I go to school now with our limited income, Marv's schedule, and no family for free babysitting?

A few days later, my inside jitters expanding exponentially, I called another conference. I told Marv I needed time to think. And to think, I needed to get away. To leave. To take a break from him and the kids. He said nothing, his face tight. He clearly didn't understand. How could he, when I didn't understand myself? He left the house, drove to the bank, and came home with a hundred dollars. "You can go Saturday. I'll have a few days free to take care of the kids."

We climbed upstairs to bed, saying nothing, my lungs ready to explode.

Backing out of the Riverdale driveway, I wondered where I'd go. I hadn't planned that part. I only knew I had to go. I turned south. Reaching Route 30, I turned west, toward Joliet. I'd never been there. As I pulled out into the openness of farmland, I felt a slight lessening of the pressure in my chest. I took a deep breath. I felt—I searched for the right word to describe the feeling—free. Free from what? Free from my little ones dependent on me for hugs, chocolate chip cookies, and dry pants? After I'd wanted them so badly, how could that be?

Meandering through the farmland, I turned up the radio. A voice announced Ray Stevens' "Everything is Beautiful." I knew what was coming, a favorite Sunday school song. My eyes watered. "Jesus Loves the Little Children." In no time, tears streamed down my face. I could barely see the road, seeing only the laughing eyes of my towheaded children. What kind of mother would leave her family?

I couldn't see. I pulled over onto the shoulder and sobbed. An ocean needed to be emptied. The song played on. The sun beat on the dashboard. The restlessness in my stomach heaved like waves in a storm-tossed Atlantic.

If I couldn't find peace, I'd never be able to go back.

My tears slowing, I eased back onto the pavement. The two-lane road curved through low rolling hills. Driving past a large white farmhouse and weathered red barn, I glanced down long furrows of newly planted fields, stretching into the sun-filled sky. Where did they lead?

The fields held hope. Something planted has to grow. Grow—a magic word.

I wasn't growing. Not in my mind. Not enough. I had to find a way to grow, a way to find peace. And I only had a few days.

About a half hour, or maybe an hour, into the drive, a sudden tiredness hit me. A sign for a roadside motel, about a dozen units with outdoor entrances, caught my attention. I turned off and checked in. "License plate?" asked the old woman in a plaid housedress, doubling as desk clerk.

"I don't know. I'll have to go out and look." Marv had filled out the registration form the few times we'd stayed at motels. The only numbers that came to mind were my kids' heights and weights.

"That's okay." Her eyes narrowed. "You staying alone?"

I thought I saw a sneer. "Yes," I said, wondering if she thought I'd be sneaking a male friend into my room later. For a second, the thought made me smile. What would she think if I said, "No ma'am. I'm running away. I don't want any guests."

As I opened the door to the room, the smell of musty carpeting reminded me of the one-room cabin where Marv and I had stayed on our honeymoon in Ludington, the place where I took a picture of our newly ringed hands, mine over his, on the white chenille bedspread.

Was I the same person?

After I locked the door, I scanned the room—knotty pine walls, double bed with faded rib cord spread, bedside table, nicked-up walnut dresser whose drawers didn't close. I started to cry again. I slid off my shirt and shorts and sat on the edge of the bed to take off my tennis shoes. Looking up, I saw myself in white cotton bra and panties framed in the dresser's mirror. But the eyes, my eyes were the saddest I had ever seen on myself—vacant, and underlined in black.

The person in the mirror was a stranger.

I put on my nightshirt, rolled back the limp bedspread, curled into fetal position, and bawled until I was dry. When I awoke, it was dark. Teeny slits of neon cut between the Venetian blinds. I turned on the lamp on the bedside table. A small clock read 9:00 p.m. I dressed and drove down the road to a diner. I was hungrier than I ever remembered being, but nothing on the menu was appealing. Eventually, I ordered a hot pork sandwich, which came with mashed potatoes swimming in gravy and a slice of red crabapple alongside. The white bread, the potatoes, the warm gravy all felt like comfort foods. A few truckers talked in low tones in a corner. A waitress dressed in turquoise offered me coffee. The jukebox played Pat Boone's "A White Sport Coat and a Pink Carnation." I finished the whole sandwich, sopping up the last of the gravy with a soggy crust of the bread.

As I wiped my mouth, I still felt totally empty, as if a crater had replaced my insides.

Turning back onto Route 30, I spotted a sign for a bowling alley in the distance. *Why not*, I thought. *I am free, I don't need a babysitter.* So I went bowling. Alone. At ten o'clock at night. No one was in the adjacent lanes, not a sound besides my own footsteps. Bending forward, I threw the ball fast—*kersmash* against the world. I got a few spares. I laughed; there were no league members to impress now. I tried to remember how to keep score. When we were dating, Marv kept score.

Marv. I couldn't believe I'd left him. Or my kids. Nausea welled up. The heavy smell of beer from guys at the bar followed me out to my car.

The next morning, a sharp sun peeked through the blinds. I felt rested, better. But now what? I dressed, checked out, and headed west, farther west. Some time later—ten minutes, an hour?—the farmland on the right side of the road butted up against a large clump of trees, like the grove just south of Marv's hometown in Minnesota. Spotting an entry road, I slowed down, and turned cautiously between the trees. The road soon ended on a small grassy clearing. I parked and moseyed down a dirt path into the dense woods. The sound of rushing water pulled me farther down the path. I came upon an opening that overlooked a shallow rolling stream. Birds swooped about, having choir practice. I sat down on a large log, dug my heels into the ground, and breathed in the scent of fresh earth. The sun touched the top of my head. Staring down into the clear ripples of water, I prayed, *God, if you see me here, help me. I can't figure this out by myself.*

It seemed like I sat on that log for hours. It got hotter. I got hungry. I looked up at the sun beyond the fresh leaves on the tall branches, painfully aware of the silence. "Be still and know that I am God" flashed through my mind. Then I heard a deep voice say, "Call Kay." Kay, my nurse-sister, my mentor, living in Toledo.

The voice had been male. Clear. I spun around but saw no one. Spooky.

Feeling lighter, I scurried up the path to my car and headed back east. Toward home. Maybe Kay could help me sort myself out. When I got close, I felt the restlessness, like the carbonation of Coke, zinging through my arteries again. Solving my unrest wasn't going to be that easy. I could not simply go home and call Kay. I wasn't ready to go home.

Spotting a phone booth at a gas station, I stopped, pushed open its bi-fold door, and dialed "0" to make a collect call. While the phone rang, traffic piled up at the nearby light. Maybe a church had just let out. It was noon. Parking lots of the few surrounding office buildings were vacant. From the station window, an attendant watched me, perhaps relieved that he didn't have to come out and pump gas. Kay answered. She accepted the charges.

"Kay," I said, my voice breaking.

"My dear, what's wrong?"

I couldn't talk.

"Take your time." Her calm voice slowed my internal Coke race.

I spilled out my story in choked pieces: "Walls closing in…Marv… motel…what now…."

She listened. "Do you feel safe?" What was she getting at? "Are you willing to call Marv?" When she seemed convinced I would call Marv, she let me hang up, but not before she made me promise I'd call her back if I couldn't reach him or if I needed something else.

When Marv answered, I cried.

"Go to Dr. Sanderson's," he said firmly, before I could say anything. "I called him yesterday. He knows you left. I'll call him now. He's waiting for a call…from either one of us."

I pulled back onto the main road. In my mind, I saw Jon building "tall towers, Mommy" with the bright blocks I'd plowed through to leave, Kathleen crawling across the green carpeting at her jet-fast speed, giggling as she spread her fingers to make Jon's tower go "boom." Marv sat next to them in the black recliner, scanning the *Sun Times*. Then the kids shimmied up on his lap, each one snuggling behind a hugging arm.

When I got to Dr. Sanderson's office, Marv was standing in the parking lot next to our old yellow station wagon. His tan stood out against his rust-colored T-shirt. As I pulled next to him, I felt his eyes search mine. Here was the man I'd met the first day of college, the man I'd married three years later—the day after I'd graduated from nurses' training—the man who'd played the game of temperature charts with me and fathered my children. The man I'd left.

He opened my car door and held out his arms.

As I stepped out, my body began to tremble. Burying myself into his embrace, I felt the strength of his arms, the softness of his shirt, the warmth of his cheek. And the familiar, comforting smell of Old Spice.

Six

TIME-OUT

*I*n Dr. Sanderson's office, the one lamp cast a soft glow on our faces as the three of us sat in a circle on leather easy chairs. Between sobs, I stammered out the story of my twenty-four hours on the run. As I talked, I read terror in Marv's eyes. What had I done to him? What could I do to fix it? What could I do to fix me? After an eternity-long pause, I said, "I know I can't go home. Not yet." I leaned over my lap, put my head in my hands, and wept again. I looked up. "I don't know where to go…we have no family around. My friends would never understand…."

There was a long silence.

"Do you think you should go to a hospital?" Dr. Sanderson asked in that caring tone he'd used often.

Hospital! Why would I go to the hospital just because I was feeling hemmed in at home? Hospitals were for sick people. I was not sick.

I tried to think, but my head felt like it was smothered in a pillow. I needed help. But a hospital? Who would take care of Jon and Kathleen? Sitters were hard to find even for short spans of time.

Feeling helpless, I looked at Marv, his face carved in lines of concern. "We'll do whatever you want, honey," he said.

Honey. His usual name for me. He rarely called me by my name.

What did I want? I wanted this unrest to disappear. Gulping for air, I searched my blurry mind for answers. None came.

Turning to Dr. Sanderson, I said in the tiniest voice possible, "Yes, I think I need to go to a hospital." I could not believe I had said those words.

"Where would you like to go?"

"Not around here," I managed to say. I didn't want to take the risk of seeing any nurse I knew. I thought of Kay. I looked at Marv. "How about calling Kay?"

Taking her number from his pocket, Marv stood, reached over to Dr. Sanderson's desk, and dialed. I wondered why he had her number.

"Kay, me again." So he had called her. Naturally he would think I might have contacted her. "Would it be possible for you to arrange an admission for Lois in Toledo?"

A heavy silence hung in the room as Kay responded to Marv. I felt as if they were having a conversation about a stranger. A former patient of mine, perhaps. I could not will myself to speak. My body sank farther into the chair.

"Okay. Could you make arrangements to take care of Jon and Kathleen, too? I have finals…also have to finish a paper yet before graduation."

More silence. I glanced at Dr. Sanderson. His expression was warm, genuine, accepting. I wanted to hug him. I wanted him to hug me. I wanted him to rescue me from myself.

"Okay," Marv said, "we'll go home, get packed up. We should be there in about five hours."

Marv put the phone in its cradle and turned to me, "It's all set, honey." He came toward me. I rose slowly and collapsed, crying, in his arms.

I don't remember the trip to Toledo. I probably tried to act normal—pointing out the pigs, cows, and horses to Jon as he stood in the back next to Kathleen in her car seat. I likely passed them Sippy cups of orange juice and Tupperware tumblers of Cheerios. I'm sure Marv and I tried to talk a little. I don't remember arriving at my sister's or Marv leaving later that night without us.

My first recollection after leaving Dr. Sanderson's office is the bang of the locked door behind me the next morning. My admission was now real. Behind the glass windows of the nurses' station, a nurse awaited Kay and me. I saw a white cap, a white uniform, a slight smile. "We're expecting you." She swung through the half-door of the nurses' station. "Follow me."

We were standing in the dayroom—a large square tiled room with a row of windows on the far wall letting in the morning sunshine. The room was empty, except for a row of vinyl-upholstered armchairs under the windows and a few scattered square tables surrounded by straight chairs in the center. Patients must have been at breakfast. I heard muffled voices off to my right and smelled oatmeal. We strode through the dayroom and turned left down a long hall, then a quick left again into a private room.

I stood, as if anesthetized, in the doorway. Straight ahead, I saw a small window. To my left, in a small alcove, a bed made with stark white linens. Was this me standing here? If not me, then who was it?

"Put the gown on—opening in the back," the nurse said, pointing to a million-times-washed patient gown on the bed. "Your clothes go in the closet. Don't leave any money here." She left, business-like, her slight smile still stuck on her face.

Kay stood at the foot of the bed while I robotically removed my cotton-knit

Bermudas and T-shirt. The aroma of starch and disinfectant clashed with the smell of my Tide-washed clothes as I handed them to Kay. She turned and hung them in the closet while I put on the gown, reaching behind me to tie the three strings down the back. No wonder my patients had problems tying the middle string—too low to reach from my neck, awkward to reach from behind my waist.

A recessed light in the tall ceiling remained unlit. The morning sun seemed to have hidden outside the window, sensing the sadness of the day.

Standing barefoot on the cold tile floor, I clutched the gown around me to keep from shivering. Kay turned back to me. Her eyes looked as though she was struggling not to cry. She took a few steps forward. I wilted into her arms. "To think it would come to this," I said, fighting back tears of my own.

I turned quickly, pulled back the stiff top sheet and limp cotton spread, crawled into bed, buried my face in the pillow, and shimmied on my stomach to get warm. The grainy texture of the hospital sheets grated across my arms. The nurse came back in. "I have a shot the doctor ordered. It will help you relax." I felt a prick in my left hip. She said to Kay, "You will need to leave soon. You may come back in three days. Rules."

What was the med? I hadn't asked. Kay leaned over and whispered, "I'll come back as soon as they let me. Don't worry about the kids. Just take care of yourself."

I felt a pat on the shoulder and heard the door shut. My head started to feel woozy. Then, as if an angel said it was now okay, a new ocean of tears began flooding my cheeks. Propping myself up on my elbows, I groped for the small gray box of hospital tissues on the bedside stand. I ripped the box open, grabbed a handful, and smashed the coarse wad against my drowning face.

While I wept, my body slipped slowly into a wide-open space. Into a mist. A thick gray mist. No walls, no floor. Nothing to contain me. I put my face in my hands and prayed, *God, don't let me explode into nothingness.* I sensed Marv's eyes, consumed with fear and helplessness, following me down my descent. Cries for "Mommy, Mommy, Mommy" echoed in my new darkened space. For the first time in my life, I felt blackness—heavy, suffocating, infinite.

As I struggled to breathe, I faded into sleep.

A repeated bang on the door woke me up. Where was I? Smelling bacon, I opened my eyes to a white bed in a white room with sun trying to come in a small window. A nurse entered, carrying a covered tray. "Time to wake up. It's Wednesday.

You've slept since Monday morning. Here's your breakfast."

Placing the tray on the overbed table, she said, "Eat up. We're taking a walk on the grounds in an hour. You're expected to come along. Rules." She smiled. "Enjoy your breakfast."

So there I sat in a hospital bed wearing a colorless patient gown and wolfing down dry scrambled eggs and cold toast in a room reminding me of a plastic igloo. I blinked a few times, shook my head to loosen a light fog, and realized I felt more relaxed and rested than I had been in months. Maybe all I needed was a mom's retreat.

The nurse reappeared. "Your doctor's here." Who was my doctor? I didn't remember Kay telling me. "Follow me. He sees his patients in an office right down the hall."

I spotted a fresh pack of linens on the chair by the door. Taking a clean gown from the top of the stack, I shook it open and put it on backwards—ties in the front—fashioning a robe of sorts to keep me covered. I was not used to meeting doctors on hospital wards out of white uniform. And certainly not without wearing underwear.

A patient's chart lay open on the office desk. My eyes zeroed in on the face sheet. My name, a diagnosis. Me, the nurse-mom who had "the problem that has no name," now had a name for it—anxiety. I don't remember my reaction to seeing that diagnosis on the page.

"What's been happening?" said the salt-and-pepper-haired man who looked like Groucho Marx.

In the five minutes he allowed me, I summed up my past few months of feeling hemmed in; my visits to Dr. Sanderson; my wish to go back to school; my running away; my return to Dr. Sanderson; my husband contacting Kay, my nurse-sister who must have called him about me.

I felt distanced, as though I were giving report on one of my patients.

After finishing my now cold breakfast, I dressed and headed for the day-room. Patients stood in line at the nurses' station for meds. Mostly middle-aged and older people. All looking dazed or tired. Probably hung over from meds. Their hair and clothes looked tired, too, as if they needed washing and fluffing. Aside from feeling a bit wobbly from my time in bed, my urge was to sprint to the head of the line and help dispense meds from the white soufflé cups the nurse had arranged in rows on her metal tray.

I reminded myself I was a patient: I wasn't working; I wasn't a visitor. I was here because I had hit bottom. I was here because I needed help to get up. I was here to get a grip on my restlessness, or my anxiety as Dr. Marx had called it. Or my whatever.

Looking around the room, I noticed a woman, maybe in her thirties—a little older than I—neatly dressed in plaid Bermudas and a golf shirt, sitting on a chair under the window, eyes bright and alert. I sensed she was home in her head and approached her. "Going on the walk?"

"Yes." She smiled and motioned for me to sit down.

"I'm going too. Guess I have no choice. Rules." We both laughed. I felt I could trust her. Something in the clarity of her eyes. "I'm new here." I paused. She waited. "I never thought I would end up here."

Her brown eyes sparkled. "Me either." She laughed. "Imagine. I work here. Downstairs in the office."

"You're kidding. I'm a nurse. Not here, though."

"Guess we both feel like we should be on the other side of that locked door, right? By the way, my name is Margaret."

Margaret and I became instant friends. I was enormously relieved to find someone "normal" to hang around with. During our free time in the afternoon, we sat in the sun under the windows in the dayroom and discussed life. She'd say, "I'm too busy to have a job and be a mom. I'm overwhelmed. I'm here because I needed a time-out. " I'd say, "I think I need a job, because being a mom isn't enough. I'm restless…so, I guess I needed a time-out, too, to figure myself out." I realized I wasn't going to become a bona fide women's libber; I didn't need to conduct sit-ins, stage demonstrations, or file discrimination charges. I simply needed to be more than Marv's wife, more than Jon and Kathleen's mom. I needed to be me again, whoever that was.

As Margaret and I talked, we watched the other patients stare, mumble, and wander around the dayroom. Once I said, "I guess we can be grateful our problems are not as severe as theirs." I wondered if I'd be like them someday. My dad's mother had had periods of feeling "low." I never met her; she, my grandpa, and my aunt were killed in a wintry car accident before I was born. One of my mother's sisters, a favorite aunt, was "high" at times. She was cheerful whenever I saw her. She sold Amway when it was just a soap product and hosted my bridal shower for the relatives. She had a son who alternated "high" and "low." He lived near us in Pine Rest where I worked in high school as a nurse's aide. We wouldn't see him for months at a time when he was depressed. But when he pulled out of the depression, he walked the few blocks to our house and held court, chattering nonstop at our kitchen table.

Maybe there were other family members I didn't know about.

As soon as she was allowed to visit, Kay came almost every day, either on her lunch hour or after work, wearing her uniform: a knee-length clean white dress. She joined Margaret and me in the chairs under the windows. "Jon and Kathleen are doing fine," she'd say. As I pictured them, tears came. My heart ached with wanting to hug them, feel their baby-powdered bodies shake with laughter against my chest.

One day, as she was leaving, Kay asked, "What did you decide to make in O.T. today? Yesterday, you were hammering an aluminum platter."

I smiled. "That was to wham out all my aggression. A Freudian thing." I sobered up and took a second to think. "You know how I hate crafts. You remember how I hated my oil painting classes."

"Yes." Kay laughed.

"Well, they don't let you just sit in O.T. You have to make something, so I decided to make something useful." I paused, glanced out the window at the trees, thought of Marv, cigarette poised between his right index and middle fingers. "But that was a difficult decision, because then it would be an item I'd take home. Something someone would ask me about—where'd I get it? Then, how would I explain? 'Oh, don't you know? I made it on a psych unit.'

"I'm not ready for that. But, I decided…I'd have to figure out how to handle that later. So, I'm working on an ashtray for Marv." I swallowed. "Today I pinched the top edge of the clay like you do on a pie crust." I held up my fingers to demonstrate. "Tomorrow I glaze it."

My eyes watered. I wondered how Marv was doing.

Over the nine, or maybe it was eleven, days I was hospitalized, my carbonated restlessness gradually lost its fizz. It helped to have to take care of only myself. It helped to talk with Margaret. It helped to keep my hands busy at the large tables in the sun-lit occupational therapy room. And, the medication Dr. Marx ordered—Elavil, an antidepressant—helped as it gradually kicked in.

Talking with Dr. Marx may have helped too, but I don't remember a thing he said during our five minutes each day. I sensed from him, however, that running away had not made me a serious case, that I was probably a typical unhappy housewife. Maybe he'd read Betty Friedan, too, or had a wife like me—a woman who would rather go to school than wax floors. I don't remember being discharged. I imagine it was after I had formulated my plan with Dr. Marx to go back to school and convinced him I was seeing cracks in the walls that had confined me.

Marv came to pick us up. The five-hour ride is a blur. The kids in the back seat probably giggled over patty-cake and bickered over Cheerios, and I, without question, hummed "Jesus Loves the Little Children."

And I would've told Marv my plan to go back to school, and he would've responded, "Hallelujah. Whatever it takes for you to be happy." And he would've told me about finishing up his grad school requirements and we would've talked about the paper I'd helped him with on systems theory. Where one change in a system changes the whole system. Like the mobile that used to hang above Kathleen's crib: if one of the miniature wooden people broke off, the mobile would tip and hang off-center. That's the way I felt then. By running away from Marv and my kids, I had tipped our family mobile out of kilter. I wanted it to hang evenly again.

I no longer had to run. My sense of humor was back. I felt "normal" again, whatever normal meant for a mom who had a "problem that has no name." And, over the next few weeks, to assure myself I was normal, I tapered myself off the Elavil.

At home, we made plans for Marv's graduation ceremony. We got a sitter for Kathleen. In the university gym, I sat high up on the bleachers and Jon stood on tiptoes next to me. We both searched for Marv in the procession. After what felt like days of vigilance, we spotted him, all six feet, two inches, marching down the aisle farthest away from us. "Daddy!" Jon yelled, smacking his pudgy hands together in an uneven tempo. Daddy was too far away to hear. I snapped a picture of the tall black smudge in the distance.

After the ceremony, the three of us posed for pictures. A cement-block wall forms the backdrop. Marv, striking in black regalia and mortarboard, a citron velvet hood (social work's color) draped over his shoulders, has his arms around us. I'm wearing a new navy dress with red flowers outlined in yellow, sleeveless with a miniskirt; Jon, dressed in "gwoan-up" long pants and navy T-shirt, clutches Daddy's leather-bound diploma.

At home, we took one more picture—Kathleen, in yellow sun suit, sits smiling on my left arm, dimpled fingers pinching a corner of the diploma. The sun is shining. I was thankful to be home.

And no one has ever asked about the ceramic ashtray filled with paper clips that sits on Marv's desk in our home.

PART TWO

Bachelor's

Seven

FINDING A FRIEND

'm sorry. That course is closed." The registrar's assistant, a slack-eyed teen at Thornton Community College in South Holland, stared at me across the counter. Her weary matter-of-fact tone told me she had said this phrase too many times already that morning. She clearly did not appreciate that I was not any ordinary student. My road to get there had been more arduous than many, I was sure.

I shifted Kathleen, now a toddler, on my left arm and clutched the mittened hand of Jon, a preschooler. Right after our breakfast of Cheerios and orange juice, with the usual fight over the one pink Tupperware glass, I had dressed the kids in their snow clothes (as they called them), driven ten minutes to Thornton, and tiptoed us across an icy parking lot to the registrar's office.

A glob that felt like a hunk of peanut butter lumped in my throat. "I cannot leave until I get into that course."

The preceding fall I had explored potential colleges for completing a bachelor's degree in nursing. University of Illinois, where Marv had gone, was an hour's train ride into the city—too far with my kids so young. St. Xavier, a private university fifteen miles away, was too expensive. The closest and cheapest option was Governors State University, a twenty-minute drive south. I interviewed there and found out that, in addition to the diploma in nursing I already had, I needed nine more hours of psychology and sociology courses as prerequisites.

The course that was closed, Social Psychology, was the only one offered one night a week. There was no way I could afford a babysitter to take a three-times-a-week daytime class.

The registrar's assistant shrugged. "The only thing you can do is see if the professor will let you in. He usually doesn't want an overload in his classes. He's teaching right now in a mobile unit across campus. You could try…."

The three of us sloshed across a snowy open field to a row of mobile units. "I'm cold," Kathleen mumbled through her scarf into my ear. My arm was numb from carrying her in her slippery nylon snowsuit. "Look, Mommy, my mittens are wet," Jon said, forming a snowball. "My hands are cold."

I bribed them. "We'll stop at McDonald's on the way home to warm up."

I found the right trailer and the right classroom. Through the open door, I saw the professor lecturing from his desk perch. When had teachers started sitting on their desks to teach?

Squeezing the three of us smack outside the doorframe, I motioned to him. He slid off his desk, waved to his class, and sauntered over. Staring at him, I said, firmly, "I need to take a course of yours that's closed. So I need you to sign this form." He drank in the portrait we presented. Maybe he thought of his wife and children, snowsuits, boots, the frigid weather. I don't know. But he shifted his eyes from me…over to Kathleen…down to Jon…and back up to me. He studied the plea in my eyes. Without a word, he signed my slip, turned, and loped back to his desk.

At McDonald's, I silently announced my good news to the world: *I am going back to school.* I imagined books and friends and stimulating study dates. The kids and I played patty-cake across the table. "Patty-cake, patty-cake, baker's man…" Our hot chocolate celebration heralded a new era for me: mom-as-student.

"If your kids ever get pinworms, come on over. I have plenty of medicine." My new neighbor in the townhouses pointed to a quart-jar-sized bottle on an end table next to the couch. "My kids get them all the time."

She must have seen the disbelief on my face as my eyes went from the bottle back to her dark eyes framed by a bush of matted hair that clumped on her plump shoulders. Her baggy T-shirt and pull-on slacks looked as though they'd never been washed. I shifted in my upholstered chair, imagining worms nestled in the crevices of the cushions.

"They come out at night," she added. "You can tell when the kids get them because they're scratching their butts in their sleep. So you shine a flash-light, spread their cheeks, and there they are—little white things crawling around. And, if they ever get lice…"

I had gone over with brownies to welcome my new neighbor. I came home shaken. "I can't stay here," I cried to Marv that night. "I can't have their kids playing with ours. It's one thing to study about worms in nurses' training, but I've never ever seen a case, and I don't intend my first experience to be with our own kids."

I reminded him the neighbor kids had already been over in our sandbox, sitting with their little wormy butts in our clean sand. And, they'd squatted in the tree house he'd built on top of the swing set for our kids. I hoped their mom was right, and the worms only came out at night.

After our first episode of pinworms, I became obsessed with moving. After the second, the doctor told me that Marv and I had to take the medicine, too. It wasn't enough to wash the kids' sheets and throw rugs every day, and wash all of our hands four hundred thousand times a day. I insisted we move; the neighbors weren't going anywhere, so we had to.

Marv agreed. He wasn't thrilled about taking worm medicine. He hugged me while I ranted. His territory as a probation officer now covered the far south suburbs, so he started noticing for-sale signs as he made visits to his probationers. One afternoon, good news at last. "I was in Park Forest today. I rode past a tri-level for sale with a large back yard—enough for a garden— and a huge open field behind it."

"Sounds wonderful. When can we go see it?" No more attached housing. No more fenced-in back yard. Jon was six, Kathleen was four, and we no longer needed a backyard playpen.

We moved in 1973. Our new neighbors didn't have pinworms. Or lice. They brought brownies, and there was one friend for Kathleen, two friends for Jon, and an invitation for me to join a local nurses' club. Plus, there was an eighth-grader eager to babysit.

All I needed was a friend for myself.

I first saw her red hair. Not ordinary red hair, but wild, bushy, like it was allergic to combs. Her eyes, piercing from under flyaway bangs, looked as if they'd seen Rome, London, Paris. Places beyond my new life in Park Forest, the "planned community" built to provide housing for World War II vets, made famous by William H. Whyte in *The Organization Man*. Her clothes—baggy jeans, plaid shirt, scuffed loafers—surprised me, a proud graduate of Stretch & Sew lessons.

Stopping abruptly in the doorway to that Marriage and the Family class, I straightened my homemade pink polyester pull-on pants and smoothed my blond pixie bangs. Suddenly, my Peter Pan-collared blouse felt too snug around my neck, and my white tennis shoes—I'd never owned a pair of loafers—looked way too clean.

"Red Hair" could be the friend I wanted. A friend with an insatiable mind for learning. Maybe Red Hair was a nurse like me. She looked my age. I wondered if she had taken classes before to spice up the housewife restlessness.

As I paused in the doorway to the classroom, Red Hair's eyes locked onto mine. I needed to meet her. Did I have the courage? Conventional me? I craved eccentricity in my tranquil thirty-something life. I'd never known anyone with wild red hair. I knew she had potential. So it was now or forever hold your peace—as my sisters and I used to say in a fight.

I headed toward her seat in the middle of the room—as determined as if I were the gingerbread woman on my way to Candy Land's castle—and sat down right in front of her. Flipping around, I said, "Hi, my name is Lois."

Red Hair searched my eyes and said, "My name is Marianna," dragging out her As like they do on the East Coast.

She seemed hesitant, but at least she'd responded.

"I haven't taken any courses before in Marriage and the Family." I rattled on, thrilled to have her attention. "I hope I learn why I married the guy I married! Some days we wonder. And I'm the baby of a family of five kids, and my brother and sisters tell me I'm a spoiled brat. So maybe I'll be able to tell them a thing or two."

Marianna deadpanned, "I'm an only child. I'm naturally spoiled."

I couldn't read her. Was that humor? The teacher called the class to order. I could hardly wait for the break.

"Why are you taking this course?" I asked.

"As a prerequisite for finishing a bachelor's degree," she said, starting a staccato conversation.

"Me, too. You a nurse?"

"Yes."

"Me, too. When did you graduate?"

"1962."

"Me, too! Where from?"

"Out east. A diploma school."

"Me, too. But in Michigan. Got kids?"

"Yeah, two. A boy and a girl."

"Me, too."

Marianna was a city girl. I was small town. She had moved recently from the University of Chicago area to a suburb near mine. She was Polish-Italian

Catholic. As a Dutch Protestant who had lived a sheltered life in a parsonage, I fantasized about city adventures into polkas, pastas, and cathedrals.

After class, Marianna said, "See you next week! Maybe we could make arrangements to take our kids to the Ella Jenkins concert together."

I'd never heard of Ella Jenkins. Elated, I danced home and hugged Marv. "I think I found a friend! Someone like me!" He grinned, suspiciously. I could read his happiness for me in the quirky grin. The next morning at breakfast, Jon and Kath sipped their orange juice in hushed silence. Each had their own pink Tupperware tumbler. A neighbor, observing their ongoing fights, had given me the pink one from her set. I made an announcement: "Guess what! Mommy's found another mommy who wants to go to school."

They didn't seem to care. I ruffled up my pixie-cut hair to make myself look a tad wild and said, louder, "After school today, we're going to the mall. Mommy needs new clothes, maybe even shoes like Daddy's that you put pennies in."

I'd dress like Marianna. I would not look like a Stretch & Sew housewife. I'd be hip.

Eight

DIPLOMA MENTALITY

arianna threw me an irreverent glance. We were in for trouble, thirty-four-year-old nurses, wives, and moms, acting like junior-high girls in their first birds and bees lecture.

"The notion of theories explaining nursing practice—like those explaining behavior in psychology—is fairly new in our discipline," the rounded-at-the-bottom, gray-haired teacher droned. "So those of you who are older diploma grads probably haven't been exposed to theories of nursing."

That described us. But as nurses who had practiced competently for years without theories, we, in 1976, doubted the usefulness of this course, my sixth nursing course at Governors State University. Marianna raised her eyebrows as if to say, "This is certainly ridiculous."

"We will begin with Dorothea Orem's self-care deficit theory of nursing. We'll first talk about the concepts of self-care deficit, self-care agency, and therapeutic self-care demand."

Deficit sounded like the national debt. Agency reminded us of insurance. Therapeutic did not fit with demand. Marianna started to giggle. I responded likewise. We didn't come back to school to learn worthless information like this.

Reading word for word from lecture notes, the teacher continued her monotone: "If a patient does not have enough self-care agency to meet his therapeutic self-care demand, he will experience a self-care deficit. And it is this self-care deficit that makes a patient need a nurse. Simply put, when the client's self-care agency, S-C-A, is less than his therapeutic self-care demand, T-S-C-D, there will be a self-care deficit, S-C-D."

Marianna's shoulders began to bob violently against mine. Her laughter was like a contagious disease and I caught it. We grabbed tissues to mop up our faces and muffle our out-of-control gasps. With the teacher still staring down at her notes, Marianna lifted a sopped tissue from her face, turned to me, and, whispering, gulped, "I'm glad…I finally know…why patients need nurses. Why they need us."

Barely able to speak between guffaws, I whispered back, "Yeah, it's great to know, finally, what we're all about. Especially in language no patient will ever understand."

For my first meeting with my advisor in her closet-sized faculty cubicle, I squeezed my size eleven self next to her (much) larger presence. There was no room to pivot or sneeze. "You have electives to play around with here," she said. "You can either bunch them to make a minor, or take a mixture of courses with no goal in mind. But, if you even have an inkling you'd want to teach someday, I recommend you make your electives count and get a minor in education."

I had to laugh. Wouldn't my mother like to hear this recommendation? I had no idea what to say, so I said, "I like the idea of taking a mixture…because a lot of things interest me. But, being mostly a mom and housewife the past thirteen years, I haven't thought much beyond getting back to school."

"Have you ever considered being a teacher?"

"Oh no. Too many teachers in my family—my mother, two sisters, a brother. I hate grading papers. I had to do that all the time with my mother. I'm here simply to learn." I thought of adding that I'd graduated from mixing up pudding at my kids' co-op nursery school and now wanted to stir up my mind, but I kept quiet.

"Then you should become a teacher," she insisted, kindly. "We'll plan your course of study to include the education courses for a minor. You won't be sorry that you'll have a specific body of knowledge, rather than a little of this and a little of that."

I didn't know enough about the other electives to argue. And I did like the notion of having expertise in an area, so I followed her plan, figuring I could change it later.

In my first education course, one that addressed teaching patients, we never opened the book. The teacher, new in 1977 to this university in the cornfields south of Chicago, announced on the first day of class that she had examined the curriculum and could not believe there was no module on communication.

"How many of you had the theory and practice of communication in your basic programs?"

None of us raised our hands.

"How have you been talking with patients when you know nothing about it? Didn't you learn how to give baths, enemas, injections?" She snapped her head left to right in front of us, catching us each in the eye. My eyes fell on the cleavage showing beneath her sheer white nylon blouse. Her voice rose. "Surely, you all learned how to start IVs, suction trachs, resuscitate patients."

Nodding in agreement, we sat silently, hoping she'd make a point.

"You've learned tasks that you perform on patients, but you never learned how to talk with them, professionally. Incredible! Starting next week, you will learn. You must buy a new text that I've ordered. Be prepared to pick partners next week and spend our three-hour class sessions participating in communication exercises."

I filed out of class, never questioning the change of course.

The following week I fussed with my pencil as I sat in the corner of a large classroom with a classmate, my pseudo-patient, from the city whom I'd never met. I was oblivious to the other students coupled around the room. Using my best newly learned introduction and open-ended question techniques, I said, "Good morning, Carolyn. My name is Lois Roelofs, your nurse on this shift. What is on your mind today?"

"I'm scared to death. I'm having nightmares." Her large black eyes matched her black slacks and blouse. "A few weeks ago, after I worked a PM, I climbed the stairs to my fourth floor apartment and found my husband dead."

What a joke! What an imaginative partner. What a good story she'd cooked up on command. I did a half-chuckle. She did not share my amusement.

"You're not telling me the truth, are you?" I stammered, wishing I could hide myself in my backpack on the floor beside me. No answer, "Well, are you?"

"Yes, I am."

Blank as my new notebook, I did not know how to respond. My cheeks felt hot. The other class members, engrossed in their interactions, did not notice us as I stumbled over inadequate words. I realized I had to hit my new book harder and take it seriously. I had to learn the "techniques of therapeutic communication"—effective ways to respond to patients. "Please tell me more," or "You must be frightened," or "I can imagine this is a very difficult time for you." And how to use silence, to say nothing.

And I had to unlearn the "blocks"—responses that didn't respect the patient's feelings—that had become habit. "I know what you mean," or "A lot of people feel this way," or "You have such a nice family to support you."

Over many weeks, my communication partner emptied her heart to me. I got to know her as a person—her fears of raising children alone in the city, her anxieties entering her apartment at night, her hopes for a safe future. I had plenty of time to use my newly learned "therapeutic communication techniques." I learned how well they could "work" to create an effective dialogue with a patient.

I got hooked.

My Thursday morning home visit felt like Sunday because I wore my new navy flats and the navy slacks of my Easter suit. The visit was for the first course I'd ever taken in community health nursing. It was the first time I'd ever been required to see patients in their homes. It was my first time not to wear whites. As I rang the doorbell in my Sunday clothes, I felt as though I should be carrying a plate of brownies.

"You're from the agency?" Ray Hart asked as he opened the door. "She's in the back. Follow me."

His wife, Jenny, lay dying in their enclosed back porch, the only room that could hold the hospital bed. After he introduced his wife to me, Ray Hart walked out. He needed a break from his twenty-four-hour vigil. "Two hours, right?"

"Yes," I said. "I'll be here for two hours."

The house smelled of pink roses, burnt toast, and the heavy sweet human odor of impending death. I placed my black bag of nursing supplies on a floral tray table. It looked spotless—too clean to dirty up with newsprint from the newspaper I'd been taught to put beneath my bag.

I didn't need any equipment, but, out of habit, I took out my stethoscope and wore it necklace-style. A Sprague-Rappaport. Top quality. My first. I'd always used a stethoscope supplied by work—one hung over the top rim of a blood pressure machine. Now I proudly owned my own.

Looking for a place to sit, I pulled up a webbed, orange-striped lawn chair to the bedside. "Mrs. Hart? My name is Lois Roelofs. I'm a registered nurse going back to school for a bachelor's degree. Right now I'm working out of your home health agency and will be spending the next two hours with you."

I said no more.

"Call me Jenny." In short phrases with labored breaths and frequent fade-out naps, she told me about her monthly pinochle club that had met since high school. The church choir taping Handel's "Hallelujah Chorus" for her. Her garden that used to be full of tulips this time of year. Her mother who died of cancer last June at eighty-five. The pink roses from a former biology student. Her fortieth wedding anniversary. The neighbors' casseroles for Ray. Her life-long habit of scraping blackness off her toast. Her embarrassment when Ray needed to clean her. Her sadness at leaving Ray behind. Her pain.

My eyes rested on Jenny while I wondered how I would spend the time. My fingers played church tent with each other. They tapped my lap without a task to do. They discovered my stethoscope and found a new place to fumble. This time I knew what to say, or, more correctly, knew what not to say.

Jenny's gaunt eyes stared past me at her unplanted garden. "Ray's too busy to keep it up."

I listened. Now and then, I would nod, say "uh-huh," squeeze her hand lightly.

For the first time in my career, I practiced nursing without needing to perform a procedure with my hands that physically invaded the patient. No medication, no blood draw, no dressing change. Not even a bath, bedpan, or back rub. Only me, learning to use myself as my own best tool. Learning how to listen. Learning when to respond. Learning what words to use.

I thanked God that a teacher had shown up in my life who knew we needed to learn therapeutic communication skills and, when she discovered the subject missing from the curriculum, had boldly inserted it into her assigned course.

"Yoohoo! I'm home." We could hear the front door banging.

"Is it two hours already?" I asked.

Ray, grinning in the doorway, repositioned his load of Sears, Jewel, and Ace Hardware bags. He'd been to Park Forest Plaza. "Got us lots of goodies, honey," he said, swinging packages toward Jenny. "We're gonna have us a date tonight. First, there's a new nightgown. Soft the way you like it…."

Jenny smiled weakly and attempted to raise her arm. Ray grabbed it and bent down to kiss her on the forehead. I could see Jenny pull strength into her smile.

Watching from my lawn chair, I told myself what a blessed morning I'd had. Almost as if my Easter clothes had really taken me to church.

The other courses I took for my education minor never taught me *how* to teach. I did learn how students process information, how to develop a curriculum, and how to analyze the contents of a nursing curriculum, but exactly how to (or how not to) approach students in the classroom, I learned by example.

In the community course where I'd met Jenny Hart, about thirty of us were jammed in a deep narrow classroom with no windows. The teacher stomped in late and, without looking at us, slammed a stack of books on the desk in front of the room. One by one they slid on imaginary stair-steps to the floor. Raking her fingers through her hair, she yelled, "One of you has made an agency visit to the Park Forest Health Department, without permission, and ruined, absolutely ruined, our chances of ever sending students there. We don't have a contract with them for clinicals, and they were incensed that a student of ours simply walked in and started asking questions."

Sitting dead-center, I felt my entire body stiffen. I'd made that visit. Alone. To get a brochure on their services for my community assessment paper. Before I flew into "fight or flight" mode, I reminded myself that I was thirty-five, for Pete's sake. Why was I letting this woman tyrannize me? But that classroom was not my kitchen; she was in charge, not me.

I figured I'd dealt with enough temper tantrums at home, I should be able to handle this situation. So, after class, I found the teacher in her cubicle and calmly confessed that it was I who'd caused the ruckus. She seemed relieved that I'd not had an ulterior motive.

A few classes later, she ranted about another serious problem. "I'm shocked at your community assessment papers. If you think you're ever going on to grad school, you're never going to make it with papers of such shoddy quality. If you even think you want to go, make an appointment to see me so I can tell you what you did wrong."

I made an appointment. Huddled together once again in her modest faculty cubicle, she taught me that when her directions for a paper include a long list of items to be addressed, I must address every item, not just nine out of ten, or nineteen out of twenty. I learned when I write percentages—thirty percent of the people are African-American, fifty-eight percent are Caucasian, and twelve percent are Other—these percentages mean nothing, absolutely nothing, without the corresponding numbers. Are there twenty people or 200 people or 2,000 people?

I never made these mistakes again—not in anything I wrote for work, for school, for home. Not even in grocery lists, family letters, or love notes to my husband.

She took one last shot at us. "Most of you are diploma grads. You got your education in a hospital, not in a college. You were socialized into acting like diploma grads. Into thinking like diploma grads. Into being diploma grads." Her tone made it sound like I had every right to be ashamed of my former education. "And, at the rate you're going, you'll have a diploma mentality for the rest of your life."

I shuddered at this shocking thought. Not me. If a diploma mentality—if being "trained" in a hospital, rather than being "educated" in a university—was such a despicable disease, I wasn't going to have it. I'd get the professional mentality of my bachelor's degree right away. I'd remember that my learning now had been based on theory or research. I'd remember that my practice, instead of being "dependent" on doctors, could now be viewed as "collaborative" with them or "independent." I'd learned well that I, as an Orem self-care deficit theory convert, could be needed by a patient, regardless of the doctor. I could practice autonomously. Yes, indeed, this notion was entirely new to me, a diploma grad used to following doctors' orders, even calling a doctor for a shampoo order if my patient wanted his hair washed.

The teacher made her point. But I felt vulnerable, belittled, and a tad stupid.

So, even though I had no formal course in *how* to teach, I learned how *not* to. Don't accuse. Don't intimidate. Don't threaten. I began to see that an effective teaching style resembled what I'd learned with therapeutic communication skills: listen, affirm. Create an atmosphere that encourages openness, instills confidence, and promotes self-esteem.

I didn't guess then I would need to develop my own teaching style very soon.

Nine

BREAKING THE MOLD

'll show you where the coffee pot is." Dr. Crow, my children's pediatrician, had greeted me with a smile and was now giving me a tour of my new job at the new HMO where he now worked.

I wondered why I needed to know the location of the pot. I didn't even drink coffee.

"There's the pot, and here's where we store the coffee and the filters," he said, motioning toward the bottom drawer of a cabinet in a storage room.

"I don't understand." Orientation to EKG machine, yes. Immunization schedules, yes. Pap smear equipment, yes. But coffee, no.

"You can make the coffee first thing when you get here at five," he said, clearing his throat. He adjusted his perfectly straight striped silk tie that stuck out between the collar edges of his starched white lab coat.

Smoothing the mock-turtle neckline of my knit Stretch & Sew uniform, I asked seriously, "What time do you start?"

"Four," he said, with a questioning look.

"You can make the coffee then. I start at five. Besides, I don't drink it. I don't make it." I laughed. "Don't even know how to work this newfangled Mr. Coffee pot. The one my husband uses at home is an old wedding present—a Farberware stainless-steel twelve-cupper."

Dr. Crow stammered, "I guess I'll make it then. I'm used to the girls making it, though."

I guessed he didn't catch on, but I was not a girl. I was a woman, a wife, a mother, and a nurse. And I'd read Betty Friedan! I did not make coffee for anybody. But, I wasn't Betty Friedan, and I thought it best not to say these words aloud. I didn't understand why he assumed I'd make the coffee. This was the man who'd said, "This mother stays" when the nurse at his former office tried to shoo me out of the exam room when Kathleen was two and needed stitches in her forehead. My status as a mother at that time seemed higher than my status as a nurse now.

Marianna had told me of the five-to-nine evening opening at this clinic. She worked here, and most of our classmates at Governors State were working also. Hearing their stories made me want to work again. I'd been home about three years with my kids. This was my first opportunity to work outside a hospital. Housed in a converted apartment, the clinic's living room became the waiting room, the kitchen was the lab, the bedrooms were the exam rooms and X-ray. Simply swinging open the outside door made my body tingle with anticipation.

After my orientation to the coffee I never made, I spent my evenings with Dr. Crow measuring babies, giving immunizations, teaching moms safety tips and feeding instructions. Now and then, he'd wink and ask, "Would you like a cup of fresh coffee?" And I'd think, *Hurrah, my first attempt at a "collaborative" practice. Even if it only involved making coffee.*

I also worked the ob-gyn side. Other than my own two pregnancies and deliveries, I had no OB experience. "This schedule is an outrage, an insult!" I protested to gray-haired Dr. Bender one busy evening.

"What do you mean?" He spoke in his grandfatherly gentle tone.

"We schedule ob-gyn patients every fifteen minutes. That is not enough time to take a history, take vitals, and do a pap smear. We need time to listen to these women. They shouldn't have to be herded through here like cattle."

"Guess you wouldn't want to work in my other office. We schedule two patients every fifteen minutes." He chuckled.

"*Two?* How on earth do you do that?"

"It can be done. You're being unrealistic. Someone has to pay for running the office. Who do you think pays for rent, heat, water, electricity, and telephones? For supplies, equipment, and salaries?"

"That doesn't justify shortchanging patients. They moved near here because we're close to a commuter train to Chicago. Their husbands are gone long days to work. Many of the women are anxious and depressed getting settled in their new neighborhoods. They need time to tell us their stories. They need to be seen as whole people, not only as Valium prescriptions."

Often, the women had been given Valium prescriptions when they'd seen internal medicine doctors first. I certainly could identify with their unrest and knew they needed a listening ear.

"Lois, you don't belong here." He spoke kindly, eyes twinkling as if he were encouraging a daughter. "You don't fit the mold. I can tell you'll be doing other things in your life. Something bigger and better. You wouldn't be content staying here."

You're right, I thought. *I didn't fit the happy housewife mold, and now I'm not fitting this workplace mold. It appears he's settled for how the system works, but I can't and I won't. There has to be a better way.* I started by rewriting the clinic's ob-gyn patient history form to be more comprehensive. The doctors found the information on the form helpful. I'd take the history first, and then they'd see the patient. Having the form ensured that patients got more time—on the first visit anyway. And developing and using the form gave me a taste of practicing in a "collaborative" role.

A few months later, as I sauntered toward an exam room to take a history on a new patient, Dr. Bender lunged out the door, stopping me short. Arms crossed over his chest, he said, "You take care of her. She wants an abortion. It's against my religion…. I wash my hands of this case."

Dumbfounded, it took me a few seconds to even think. In my many years of hospital nursing on medical-surgical units, I had never been faced with this situation.

Every Sunday at church I recited, "Thou shalt not kill." But didn't the patient have a right to know that her insurance at our clinic covered abortions?

Who would I find if I went into the room? A rape victim? A twenty-year-old using the recent Roe vs. Wade decision for birth control? A forty-year-old mother of five who felt she couldn't handle any more children?

I questioned my right to impose my morality on a patient. I questioned for what purpose I would make her feel guilty for her choice. At my capping in nurses' training, I had recited the Florence Nightingale pledge, promising to "devote myself to the welfare of those committed to my care." With that pledge in my heart, I'd never walked away from a patient, and I couldn't walk away now. But what did "welfare" include? Certainly not killing. But what about her circumstances—her family support, financial situation, and emotional state?

My legs felt like they were mired in mud. I tried to think clearly.

What would my ever-compassionate dad do? My dad left his family of five to pastor young men as a chaplain during World War II. My dad fed "hobos" who showed up on our parsonage doorstep asking for Greyhound bus money. My dad became an appreciated presence to his parishioners during times of loss because of his own loss of his folks and sister.

I was still alone in the hallway, struck with fear. I recalled my dad's letter to his seminary professor seeking counsel about a "forced delivery" when my mother was pregnant with me. Her doctor had advised that they might need to choose between her life and mine. After consulting with physicians, the professor replied that it would be ethically permissible to resort to a "surgical miscarriage." Even so, my folks decided to take the risk, hiring a housekeeper for the other four children and sending my mother to bed for months in the sewing room behind the kitchen of the Peoria, Iowa, parsonage. Now I, the living result of their courageous prayerful decision, was faced with helping a young woman who wanted to end her pregnancy.

Could I do this? Should I?

I forced my legs to move and knocked lightly on the door. A woman in her twenties sat hunched on a straight chair next to the desk, long hair hanging forward. I picked up her chart. "Hi, Nancy, my name is Lois Roelofs, one of the nurses here. Dr. Bender told me you want to have an abortion." I spoke quietly while I pulled my desk chair out to sit nearer to her. "Would you like to tell me about it?"

Wiping her eyes with a giant handkerchief, she stammered, "Missed one period…pregnancy test positive…a foolish mistake…no money…my parents will kill me…guy not in the picture…I can't do this alone…I'm a college student…I need help."

"Have you thought about trying to have the baby?"

"No-o-o-o," she sobbed. I handed her a fistful of tissues. "I mean, yes, I've thought about it. A lot. Stayed awake for nights trying to figure it out." She sucked in a big breath and focused directly on my eyes. "Don't try to talk me out of this. I've made up my mind. I want to go through with this. I must go through with this."

Fingering the stethoscope around my neck, I tried to think of what I should or should not say. I couldn't imagine being in her situation; Marv and I had struggled to get pregnant. At that very minute, Jon and Kathleen were home with Marv, probably eating Spaghettios and grilled cheese sandwiches cut into triangles.

I started quietly. "I've not experienced what you're going through. I don't know what it's like." I concentrated on keeping my voice calm. "But I'd like to give you choices. I will give you a phone number for a pregnancy counseling center. Whatever you decide, to go ahead with the abortion, or if you just want to talk about going through with the pregnancy, you can call this number for help." Tears stung my eyes as I reached for her hand. "And I will give you the number for our clinic downtown. Under your insurance plan, you'd go there for an abortion. But you'd come back here to Dr. Bender for follow-up care."

"Would I be able to see you, too?" she asked.

"Sure. Schedule your visit on a Monday or Thursday evening."

In silence, she followed me down the hall to the nurses' station. I wrote down the phone numbers for her and accompanied her out of the office down a short hallway to the outside door where she gave me a quick hug. Neither of us said anything. My sadness for her felt as heavy on my chest as the lead apron we used in our X-ray room.

Two weeks later, I saw her name on the appointment book. I told Dr. Bender I would see her first. When I entered the room, she sat in the same place next to the desk. Her face lighter, her hair pulled back. I greeted her, quietly, and sat down.

She reached out her hand and took mine. "Thank you." Her eyes told me the story of her relief. "I'm here for the check-up you said I should have. Then I have to get back to school."

Heading toward the next exam room, I still wondered if I'd done the right thing. And I still wonder now, but am thankful that I had the presence of mind in that tense new situation to offer the woman options.

As I saw the next patient, I wished unwanted pregnancies were a black and white issue like blood pressures. Taking vitals on a forty-ish large woman, I discovered a blood pressure of 220/150. She'd come in to see Dr. Bender for her annual pap smear. When I asked her what her normal blood pressure was, she started to cry. "I had no idea. I'm a bus driver. People with blood pressure problems can get strokes, can't they? I can't put my school kids in danger. What can I do?"

I told her we'd schedule her to see one of the internists right away. This problem was clear cut—it required no ethical decision-making—and could be addressed: diet, medication, exercise. And, thanks to Marianna for her entrepreneurial plea with the clinic's administrator to establish a "nurse visit," I told the patient we'd also schedule her to see me weekly so I could take her blood pressures and monitor her progress.

The patient smiled with relief. She didn't know this would be the first time anyone would make an appointment to see me alone. It gave me a sense of independence and responsibility, and it felt good. For HMO members, a "nurse visit" was included in their plan; private pay patients were charged five dollars. Even though it was a nominal fee, Marianna and I were thrilled with the "principle of the matter." And for the opportunity to practice in an "independent" role.

Another night I was hanging out in the lab while the tech was performing a test. "Oh no, this one's gonorrhea," she said. "Seems like I had a man last week with the same name—Spicer—and same bug." Our lab tech's eyes were intent on the microscope.

I'd assisted Dr. Bender earlier with Lucille Spicer's pap smear. I didn't know other tests had been ordered. The doctor sauntered into the tiny lab. "What's the verdict?"

"Gonorrhea."

"So how do you deal with this?" I asked him. "Sounds like it may have been her husband who was in last week for the same thing. I wonder who gave it to whom."

"Her husband got it from another woman. I checked his file."

"So what do you tell the patient?"

"That she has an infection, and she must take medication for awhile to clear it up."

"What?" I screamed in a whisper so Mrs. Spicer couldn't hear across the hallway. "You mean to tell me her husband's been playing around, and you're not going to tell her?"

"Don't you think the husband has learned his lesson? Do you want to break up a marriage?"

My brain went on a rant. Break up a marriage! Wasn't it already broken? Why must the husband be protected? Doesn't the wife have a right to know her own illness?

Enraged, I waited for him to come out of Mrs. Spicer's room. I entered, took the chart, attempted to smile, and walked her to the front desk. She greeted her husband, sitting alone in the waiting room, wearing a windbreaker and jeans. Why had he come along? "It's only an infection," she said as if to reassure him. "A couple of pills and I'll be okay."

He quickly laid down his magazine and grinned. Mrs. Spicer turned to make her next appointment. Mr. Spicer glanced at me. What could I do? There were no laws that said a sexually transmitted disease had to be reported. I couldn't make Dr. Bender talk to Mr. Spicer. I could only shoot him a killing look as I passed by to vent to Marianna working at the other end of the hall.

This is not fair, I said to myself. *Simply not fair.* I was only beginning to appreciate the enormity of each decision made in practice. I was only starting down the road that gentle Dr. Bender had traveled for many years. I didn't doubt that he made decisions that were right for him, ones I hoped and sensed that in his grandfatherly way he had agonized over. Now I would have to learn to do the same.

My student life and work life eventually collided. I approached the head nurse at the clinic when she came in to post hours. "I have a conflict coming up," I said. "One of my final courses I need to take at Governors State is offered only on Mondays and runs for eight weeks. Is there any way you could start hiring an agency nurse to fill in for this short time?"

As one of only three nurses, I'd filled in for vacations so many times that I'd often averaged twenty hours a week, rather than my assigned ten. I anticipated they'd accommodate me because I'd willingly helped them avoid the need for agency nurses. The head nurse, with a blank slate demeanor, said she'd check with the administrator. She came back to me and said I'd have to quit or not take the class.

I called the administrator.

"You were hired to work Mondays and Thursdays. Now you can't work Mondays and I've been informed there's no way to cover for you…you can file a grievance, if you wish, with headquarters at the main office downtown."

I filed the grievance. I asked Marianna if she'd go along and fight with me. She initially said yes, then, a few days later, said no. She gave me no reasons.

I was angry; I didn't understand. I drove twenty-five miles to the city alone, lost the grievance, lost the job. But I didn't want to lose Marianna as a friend, so I made up a reason for why she wouldn't want to become involved: her husband commuted to work with our administrator. We still connected at school, and our friendship continued as if nothing had come between us. Much later, she would tell me she'd always regretted not being there for me.

A classmate told me of a part-time job in a steel mill. Twelve-hour shifts, from 6:00 p.m. to 6:00 a.m. I applied, eager to work in another new environment and to learn new procedures. I treated burns with Silvadene. I irrigated eyes to flush out microscopic steel slivers. I used alcohol to wash black dust off counters and aluminum cabinets.

The best part of the night was taking a break to listen to the wiry gray-haired night foreman on his ten-minute break. He'd relax on the bench under the window across from my steel desk, place his cap on his knee, and recount story after story of years of caring for his wife with multiple sclerosis. Love filled his measured words and shone in his deep-set eyes.

As I watched the foreman, the glow of the moon would skirt his shoulder. Mysterious noises hissed from the mill through a door on my left. After ten minutes, the horn announcing break times pierced the silence. The foreman would stand to leave. "See you tomorrow night," he'd say, adjusting his cap back on his head.

I loved this man, as I did all the men who'd stop by in the dark hours of their graveyard shift and tell me scraps of their family news—a new baby with all its fingers and toes perfect, a first communion with even Aunt Josie present, a twentieth anniversary celebrated at the American Legion Hall.

I didn't miss hospital nursing at all. Going back to school had been a good thing. It had opened new opportunities. I loved "independent" practice. I no longer felt hemmed in or like I had to run away. I now had many roads to take.

June 1977. Graduation. My folks, spiffed up in new polyester outfits, came with Marv and the kids. Our little family of four stood by the small pond at Governors State for pictures. In one, Marv is smiling down at me and holding me close, his blue leisure suit accentuating his six-foot, two-inch frame. I'm clutching my diploma, and under my black robe I'm wearing a size nine sleeveless jumpsuit, black with white polka dots.

In another picture, Jon, ten, is standing on my right, wearing long checked pants with a white T-shirt. The top of his head reaches my ear lobe. On my left, Kathleen, seven, hugs my leg. Her shoulder fits snugly under my arm, wrinkling her pink and white dress. Her white kneesocks and red Mary Jane's contrast against my robe. I feel the warmth of my children's bodies next to mine. I feel good.

I wanted to hug Marv, my kids, and my diploma forever. Finally, eighteen years after graduating from high school, I'd earned my bachelor's degree, and I'd done it being a wife and a mother—and with their help! Betty Friedan had been right. I did not have to stay a trapped housewife.

What would I do next?

Decisions could wait. First, there was the church picnic, Vacation Bible School, Kath's eighth birthday party at the picnic table in our back yard, my dad's seventy-fifth birthday party at his church a half an hour away, my fifteen-year Blodgett reunion in Grand Rapids.

And the house to clean....

Ten

BLUFFING IT

*H*oney, there was an ad in the paper today for a clinical instructor at Prairie State. In med-surg." The kids had kissed Marv good night; I'd tucked them into bed on the upper level of our tri-level in Park Forest and joined Marv in the living room.

Marv put his paper down, knowing from experience that some sort of plea was going to follow my call-to-attention "honey" statement. "I could try doing what I did that last summer in nurses' training, the summer before we got married. Supervising students as they work on the floor."

"You want to try it? Go for it." He picked up his paper and resumed reading.

Why not, I thought. I'd been told by my advisor at Governors State that I could be a teacher someday with the education minor she'd insisted I take. Besides, it had been several months since I'd graduated, and I was getting bored at the steel mill. Since the community college with its two-year nursing program was only about five miles away, the hospitals where they had clinicals could be close, too. If I was lucky, Marv, in his current job as a school social worker, could get the kids off to school and I could be home before they got home.

I made an appointment with the chair, Carolyn Zimmer, and pondered my closet. My best Sunday outfit would have to do: all in brown—a floral polyester blouse, pull-on slacks, and a wool checked blazer.

"This position is primarily med-surg." Mrs. Zimmer, petite with fluffy bleached blonde hair, stared at me across her desk and did not stop to breathe. "You will spend twelve weeks at St. James Hospital right here in Chicago Heights on the fifth floor with a mixture of medical and surgical patients. You will have no more than twelve students to supervise. You will assign each student to one patient. The students give baths, do treatments, and give all medications and IVs. The most important thing for you to do is to monitor the administration of the meds and IVs—to make sure there are no errors."

She was talking as if I already had the job. I had barely sat down. Was it this easy? Have a brand new bachelor's degree, show up, and be offered a teaching contract? I suddenly felt like an old established teacher and guessed this meant I'd be grading papers, like my mother. I quickly squashed my miserable memories of helping her grade her fifth graders' math tests.

"I'm interested." I talked fast before Mrs. Zimmer could figure out I was an imposter and she would change her mind.

As she leaned back in her chair, the overhead light in the small office glared off her glasses. "Fine then. You'll be working with the sophomore teaching team. Oh, by the way, the first four weeks of each semester are psychiatric. You'll go to the state hospital about forty-five minutes south of here."

Oh no, I thought. *I can't go that far away from home. I've got kids in school. And, I can't do psych. I'm med-surg. I'd have no idea what to do with twelve students on a psych ward.* Visions of my own three-month psych experience at Chicago's Cook County Hospital in 1961 came to mind. Giving paraldehyde shots with needles so dull they took a U-turn in the patients' buttocks. Sitting with an intake patient, brought in by police paddy wagon, who put a warm cough medicine bottle into my hands, and then told me it was vomit. Watching, through a peep hole in a door to a private room, a patient restrained by leather straps around his wrists and ankles managing to line up his hand-made fecal "walnuts" on the side rail.

I remembered failing the midterm exam and being sentenced to the dark, bleak library in the nurses' dorm. As I sat there for hours while classmates were exploring the top of the Prudential Building that had opened a few years earlier in the Loop, I became convinced I'd never work in that field again. Staring at Mrs. Zimmer, I gasped, "Oh, I'm sorry. I wouldn't be at all comfortable in psych. I'm going to have to say no."

Paying no attention, Mrs. Zimmer stood up behind her desk, picked up two thick nursing textbooks, and heaved them on my arms that had involuntarily swung open.

"You'll do fine, I'm sure. I'm happy to have you join us. Thanks for coming in."

Driving home, I couldn't make sense of what had happened. All I knew for sure was that I was now, in 1978, a teacher. To celebrate, I stopped for an Arby's Junior and a mocha shake and watched the traffic on Route 30 and Western, the same corner I'd called Marv from the weekend I'd run away from home eight years earlier. My dream then of going back to school for a bachelor's degree had certainly come true. And now it had opened this new door. It seemed the corner had prospered, too. I didn't remember it being as populated with commercial buildings.

I pulled into the driveway a few minutes before our kids came home from school. Then it was back to reality—milk and chocolate chip cookies at the kitchen table; Jon, now almost eleven, and friend on the family room floor constructing villages with Lincoln Logs and his Erector Set; and Kathleen, eight, and friend playing Barbies in her room. After the kids' bedtime, I spent the evening scanning my new textbooks. For the first time, I found out what "teaching knots" in my stomach felt like. Drawing pains, similar to the pains I'd had as a young mom on no-breakfast mornings before a TOPS weigh-in. At least then, after the meeting, I'd be able to eat. Now, no food could sugarcoat these knots.

The following Monday, I met my teaching team. Maureen, a veteran teacher nearing retirement who taught psychiatric nursing, asked if I'd like to audit her class. This required extra time, but I attended because I was afraid I didn't remember enough from my diploma program. Sitting in the back row of fifty students, I was spellbound by Maureen's teaching style.

Short with gray hair, Maureen wore a stern look complemented by unexpected smiles, chuckles, and humorous anecdotes. Wearing slacks and a blouse, she paced rhythmically across the front of the classroom, interspersing lecture with acting out the behaviors common to each illness. The person with depression, for example, shuffled across the room with slumped posture, her face devoid of affect. She whispered, "I feel like no one cares about me anymore." The person suffering from schizophrenia glanced furtively around the room—suspicious that someone was watching. Then she pointed inside her mouth and said, "The FBI are hiding in this filling." The person experiencing obsessive-compulsive disorder paced the room checking and rechecking the desk, door, and window locks.

Maureen's depictions vividly portrayed patient suffering. I felt as if I were on a psych ward empathizing with patients' pain. I memorized her words and movements, never anticipating they would become part of my own teaching repertoire.

She offered to drive me to the clinical. Marv got the kids off to school, and I became Maureen's student in the car. She taught me how to bluff, an invaluable skill for any teacher. "You bluff it, Lois, you simply bluff it. Think of it. You know more than the students. They don't know you don't know—unless you tell them. Act like you're an experienced teacher; they'll never know the difference."

So bluff I did. On the first day of clinical, I had to give a tour of the building. Not having any idea what was in such a building—I'd never been in a state psychiatric facility—I was relieved to see signs projecting from the wall over each doorway. Leading my group of twelve students, I announced each sign: "This is music therapy. Patients come here to experience music as a treatment," "This is Art Therapy. Patients come here to express their feelings through art," and "This is the library. Patients can come here and read."

I was off to a brilliant start.

Then, with my dayroom keys, I unlocked a heavy door, held on to the doorknob, shooed my students inside, followed them in, closed the door, and turned the knob to make sure the door had relocked. I felt powerful with those keys; it was my first time as a nurse to have any keys other than keys to narcotic cupboards. But I quickly lost any feeling of power. The dayroom seemed to be the size of a domed football field. Ghost-like sounds echoed off its institutionally bland walls. Stark chairs and radiators lined the perimeter. Shabbily dressed people sat blank-eyed in the chairs. Others slept on the floor next to the heaters. With no confidence, I led my group through the empty center of the room—as far away from the patients as possible. To keep from hyperventilating, I kept reminding myself Maureen would come anytime I needed her. She was one minute away in a ward across a connecting dining room.

I stopped in the middle of the room, and as I turned to face my lineup of students, bedlam broke loose in my stomach. I jammed my hands in my lab coat pockets. Checked to make sure the keys were securely pinned. Swallowed.

Now what do I do? Where do we sit? What do I have the students do?

"I am Jesus Christ," a large, tall man, arriving from nowhere, yelled into my face. As I jerked back, he leaned over and planted a kiss on my forehead. "You are blessed forever."

My vision blurred. I willed blood up to my head. I swallowed the breakfast threatening the back of my throat. As abruptly as he'd arrived, he left. Bluff it, Maureen had said, bluff it. Gulping frightened breaths that sounded like panting during childbirth, I faced my lineup of twelve instant ice sculptures and said, "As we've discussed, we must be alert. We must stay calm."

I prayed for calmness myself.

On the drive home, I rambled to Maureen about my morning's experiences. One you-won't-believe-this story after another. She chuckled. "Sounds like you did a great job! I kept waiting for you to come over for help, but you never did. You survived all on your own. Welcome to psych nursing!"

That evening, I called Marianna, who was also teaching. She told me of bumbling through a dressing change with a student, and I told her about bluffing my way through the "Jesus Christ" incident. We laughed so hard we could hardly finish our stories. We'd never dreamed of ourselves as teachers.

At the end of the semester, after a more comfortable experience on a med-surg unit in a general hospital, Mrs. Zimmer called me into her office. "There's a new state law coming down that will require faculty to have a master's degree in order to teach," she said. "I think you ought to go for it. You seem to have a knack for this."

What next? I now wanted to be a teacher. I could thank my bachelor's advisor for pointing me in this direction. However, for a master's program, I had to declare a clinical specialty. And I was a med-surg nurse with this new fling into psychiatric nursing. I knew I didn't want to learn any more about bowels, lung secretions, or the circulatory route of the heart. I wanted to know more about how people respond to their illness. I wanted to know more about what to say and what not say and how to listen as they were faced with their losses. With that in mind, I could also thank the teacher in my bachelor's program for pointing me, inadvertently, through the required communication exercises, toward psychiatric nursing.

I wonder, now, what would've happened if I'd never gone back to school for my bachelor's, if I'd stayed home and continued to try sewing, bowling, painting apples. Or spending more time playing Sorry, Uncle Wiggly, or Chutes and Ladders with my kids. Or running church dinners, leading a Brownie troop, volunteering at a food co-op. No way. I couldn't have done it. Just thinking about it gives me the jitters.

While my children took piano lessons, I stole time at a nearby pancake place, Golden Bear, and studied for the Graduate Record Exam, an entrance requirement to graduate school. I relearned math ("opposite angles of isosceles triangles are equal"), refreshed my vocabulary ("cacophony"), and sharpened analytical skills ("If six women are sitting in a circle and fourteen candy bars need to be distributed evenly, what would you do?").

As I drove out of Golden Bear and crossed Western to the piano teacher's home, I hoped I'd come up with the right answers for the timed exam before the bell rang. I hoped I'd stay calm in the huge tiered cement-walled classroom downtown at the University of Illinois, Circle campus. I hoped I'd fit in, a suburban housewife and mom, on my first academic endeavor away from the comfort of my Chicago suburb and into the unknown bustle of a city campus.

I didn't have time to worry long because the kids jumped into the car (taking turns for the front seat) and regaled me with stories about learning to count aloud while playing their pieces. For my old-fashioned "one and two and three and," they were learning to say "apple, cherry, or blueberry" (or something like that; even they don't remember anymore). With a penchant for metronomes, my piano-teacher mother would've said with disdain, "What next!"

PART THREE

Master's

Eleven

MEETING SADIE

ntent on eavesdropping, I hovered by the back door that faced the driveway, the orange door I'd painted bright and glossy in a spasm of boredom to perk up our brown clapboard house. The door flashed the green smiley face: "Thank You for Not Smoking," my message to Marv that he honored in the house.

Marv, nail apron tied over his jean shorts, was standing about ten feet away with Harry, our neighbor in Park Forest. Harry, hands in his pockets, white shirt open at the throat, and balding head wet with sweat, was saying, "…good care of her, Marv. I'll come by for her at 6:20. She can walk with me to the 6:47 train. We'll get to the Loop in time for her to transfer to the 'L' and make it to her eight o'clock classes."

"Thanks, Harry. I'm sure she'll appreciate it—this is a major venture for her."

I smiled. In addition to being a housewife and mom, I soon would be a regular train commuter for the first time. The University of Illinois would be even farther away than my clinical commute for teaching. It was fun to hear Marv's happiness for my neighbor's unsolicited offer of protection.

Harry came by for me as promised at 6:20 on my first day. September 1979. As we were hoofing the mile to the Illinois Central train station in Matteson, he said, "Three of us sit in the north end of the last car, in the seats facing each other. There is room for you to join us." For the next two years, he and his fellow commuters, a man and a woman, adopted me as their safety project. While they read their newspapers, I'd review class notes.

In the underground terminal at Michigan and Randolph, I caught whiffs of coffee, donuts, and flowers. Different from the smells of Tide, CoCo Wheats, and flowering crab apple trees I'd left at home. Harry guided my arm as we zigzagged between the small stores up to the street. He taught me to be street savvy: pull a straight face, stare straight ahead, ignore the paper cup of guitar-playing panhandlers. Pointing me west toward Marshall Field's—in the direction of the 'L' to the Medical Campus, he said, "You're on your own now, Lois. Hope to see you on the 5:30. Remember we sit in the south car again."

I fell in love with downtown Chicago. Towering buildings. Rushing crowds. Honking taxicabs. I felt the excitement of being an instant transplant from Burbsville, USA. The empty streets, sprawling back yards, and one-story shopping centers of Park Forest seemed a world away.

The 5:30 train home might come too soon for me to want to leave the fun.

I passed Field's and found the State Street entrance to the underground walkway to the Blue Line. Standing tall with my ten-dollar K-Mart backpack in place, I fell into a fast-paced lineup of people. Faking confidence, I followed them into the darkened cement tunnel, paid my fare, and boarded the train that only seconds before had screeched to a halt with sounds like fingernails on a chalkboard, only worse.

I didn't dare sit down. As the train emerged out of the darkness to ground level, I stared out the window, scanning every sign for the Medical Center stop. What if I missed it? Would I know how to backtrack? Would I be late for my first day?

I hoped I'd made it on to the Blue Line. Harry had said to make sure I didn't get on the Red Line by mistake. Then I'd have to get off at the Cook County Hospital stop, and that was not a safe place for a novice to be roaming around in the city.

I made my face go blank; I didn't want anyone to see how naive, how scared, or how excited I was.

When I got to the College of Nursing at 845 South Damen, Marianna was waiting for me in the lobby. Since we'd completed our bachelor's degrees two years earlier, she'd moved west of the city, an hour away from my southern suburb, and we'd begun planning to meet in the city and do another degree together. After comparing catalogues, courses, and costs of several universities, we settled on U of I and then spent a few anxious months hoping for our acceptance.

Excited as kids trick-or-treating for Halloween candy, we scampered across the street to the Illini Union bookstore to buy our books. Armed with two paper shopping bags apiece, we returned to the College of Nursing for an orientation session. We stood first in line at the closed door of the first floor assembly hall. All of a sudden, a woman opened the door, almost uprooting us. She called out, "Please move back, everyone, and make room for the graduate students to enter."

Marianna and I backed up, allowing those behind us to enter the room. It occurred to us, at the same time, *we* were graduate students. We'd hardly had enough time, as old diploma school grads, to think of ourselves as bachelor's grads. Maybe my former professor was right: I'd have a diploma mentality the rest of my life! Trying to contain our hysterics, we joined the others.

At the end of the day, we found we each had qualified for federal grants—full tuition and $400 per month. What a relief…and a surprise after no response to financial aid applications months before. My advisor told me to thank Rosalyn Carter, the President's wife. Due to her interest in mental health, federal monies had been appropriated for graduate education in psychiatric nursing.

Now I wouldn't have to ask Marv for spending money; I hated being financially dependent. I could even buy a watch. I needed a reliable one to make my trains.

The first day of fun ended. From then on, Marianna and I were separated. She started her classes in public health nursing, and I began mine in psychiatric nursing. We even took our research courses with classmates in our own clinical specialty. But we managed to meet often: at the Union at the end of a tiring day, at Stouffer's downtown for an early morning coffee, or at Field's Ice Cream Palace for Frango mint sundaes. In the mirrored walls of the Palace, we could see our tired student eyes and matching plaid coats—hers was gray and mine was brown—as we savored the smooth chocolate and temporary respite from studying.

I dreaded research. I knew how to research information in the library for writing a paper, but I'd hated my required course at Governors State in which I thought I'd learn the process of conducting an actual research study. A diploma grad like me, never exposed to research-based nursing practice…I wanted to know what the hullabaloo was all about. I wanted to know what it actually meant to identify a researchable nursing problem, design a study, collect and analyze data, and then come to conclusions that could be used to better nursing practice.

Instead I'd learned lists of words. Crazy words that, without grasping them in context, I never comprehended at all. Words like variables—dependent, independent, and extraneous. Words like designs—experimental, quasiexperimental, and nonexperimental. Words that hadn't mixed well with my mom phrases of "Spaghettios again?" or "Your room looks so neat" or "We'll have to talk to Dad about this."

The first day in graduate research, my classmates and I flanked a rectangular seminar table in a small room of the same shape. "Let's talk about your research interests," the professor said. "What is it you want to do for your thesis?"

I'd known about the required thesis, but certainly had never seen myself as a researcher, nor had I planned on having to know what I would do for the thesis this soon. What would I say?

Going around the table, the first student said, "I want to study the adjustment response of primiparas to episiotomies."

I was impressed. She already knew what she wanted to do. It had been years since I had studied obstetrics, but I recalled this had something to do with first-time mothers and an incision sometimes made to enlarge the birth canal. Another student said she planned to study something about jeans. I fingered my Levi's under the table. Then I realized she was talking about g-e-n-e-s. I'd watched Sesame Street too long!

Panic produced my only thought for a research question: Why does a middle-aged mom ride trains to get a master's degree? Funny how I thought then that thirty-seven was middle-aged. When my turn came, words—from way back—fell from my mouth. "I'm a med-surg nurse who's always been interested in how my patients respond emotionally to their illness."

The teacher moved on to the next student. I had crossed my first hurdle.

The psychiatric nursing clinical specialty was designed to prepare us as therapists. We could choose two of three treatment modalities: group, family, and individual. I didn't see myself ever working with individuals as a therapist, so I chose group and family. They would be the most useful in the everyday life of working with students, faculty members, or patients. They should help me understand why people behave the way they do.

I did not realize I would also learn about my own behavior, my own dynamics.

The first day in the group psychotherapy course, held in a darkened videotaping room lit by spotlights, the professor stood at the head of the class. "You will learn the dynamics of group behavior through personal experience in your student group. Your chairs are arranged in a U-shape for a reason. I'll set up the video camera here in the open space to record your interactions. Then I'll leave. Each week, after the group meeting, you'll do the assigned readings, view the videotape in the fourth floor library, and analyze the groups' behavior according to what you've read."

The prof turned on the video camera and left the room. Eleven of us, strangers—one male—painstakingly progressed through stages of how groups develop. According to Tuckman's theory, we formed, stormed, normed, and performed. We mostly stormed. Along the way we discovered what roles we play within groups. I found we often reenact the roles we have within our own families. I had to dig, dig, and dig into why I behaved the way I did—the baby of a family of five children, called the "spoiled brat" by my siblings. Why did funny comments naturally pop out? Did I need to be heard? Did I need to lighten up conversations when the mood got tense? Or was I simply gifted with a sense of humor that my four siblings said skipped over them and was given to me? I'd never had to look at myself objectively before. And why was I angry that we couldn't move past our storming "power and control" stage? Did I feel superior because I was older? Did I feel wiser because I had the oldest kids? Or was I simply more experienced working within groups? In the margins of my weekly analysis paper, the prof persistently prodded me to explore my own issues as well as those of the group.

This was more than I'd bargained for in choosing this clinical specialty. Maybe learning more about communicating with patients *wasn't* my thing. Perhaps I should've been more interested in bowel movements, blood circulation, and lung secretions and gone med-surg!

After this jolt into self-awareness, the group dynamics courses grew to be favorites. Watching my own behavior in a group became second nature. Did I help the group process by being an encourager, harmonizer, or problem solver? Or did I obstruct by being a monopolizer, complainer, or moralist?

And, of course, Marv bore the brunt of my new knowledge. Why were we behaving the way we were anyway? Even though he'd been educated as a psychiatric social worker, he was not into analysis—not at home, anyway.

A subsequent course required leading a group for twenty consecutive sessions. My co-therapist Janice, the only classmate near my age, helped us gain entry into a nursing home with a psychiatric population. We screened for a group of eight members. Every week we each tape-recorded the ninety-minute session, transcribed the tape longhand—nearly wearing out the pause buttons—and analyzed interactions according to the theories we were learning.

In the group I met Sadie—in her fifties, diagnosed with schizophrenia. She marched into each group session broomstick-straight, but tilted backwards about ten degrees. Wearing white square-heeled shoes, red anklets, and a cotton floral housedress, she resembled a forties housewife in an ad for detergent. She kept us on task: if we didn't start right on time, she'd glare at Janice and me and ask in a loud staccato monotone, "What are we waiting for?"

Sadie told her history. As a young mother many years before, she'd suffered from epilepsy. Because of the lack of available treatment at the time and her uncontrollable seizures, doctors admitted her to the state hospital and much later to this nursing home. She didn't seem aware of her eccentric behavior or psychiatric diagnosis. Only the term "untreatable epilepsy" stuck in her mind.

Sadie made clear to me the effects of 1963 legislation under President Kennedy supporting deinstitutionalization of the mentally ill from state and county facilities into the community. The intent was good—remove people from warehousing environments and integrate them into communities. But Sadie's home had been the state hospital for so long that she missed her job working in the sewing room and her freedom roaming the spacious grounds. Now, with no work and neighbors who didn't want residents with psychiatric diagnoses on their streets or in their stores, she described her frustration: "What do they expect me to do? Sit outside and smell the car exhaust? I'd like to walk, but there's no place to walk. The only place you can walk here is around the building, and I refuse to do that. It would make me look like I was a dummy going round and round."

These words became the opening paragraph of my master's thesis. Unwittingly, Sadie had given me the topic that had eluded me the first day of the research course. One day in class during winter quarter, I lamented that I still didn't have a research problem I wanted to study. A classmate jumped in, "It bothers you that Sadie complains she has nothing to do. Why don't you ask older people how they'd like to spend their day?" She was right. Sadie's plight of boredom sent me to the library to study the concept of "free time" that led to my master's thesis, "Leisure Preferences of the Institutionalized Elderly."

By the end of the twenty weeks, Sadie's story had found a permanent home in my heart. I felt called on her behalf to advocate for the mentally ill. I felt sure I could do this best as a teacher. Over the years, I could tell her story to lots of students who, in their own practice of nursing, could work toward bettering the lives of those people affected by mental illness.

Apparently, I'd made an impression on Sadie as well. After the other group members left the final session, she invited me to her room and presented me with an egg-shaped vase containing a plastic red rose covered with water. As I write this, over twenty-five years later, the rose still stands on my desk and serves as a reminder of Sadie's legacy to me.

My next clinical course, family therapy, exposed me to abuse, as well as dogs, cats, and cockroaches. Janice found us a family through her contact with a rural public health department. The referral nurse, who served as our clinical preceptor, assigned us a family of four. Tom, the father, had an alcohol addiction. Dorothy, the mother, suffered from depression. And there were two children: Susie, aged nine, and Andy, four. The nurse explained that the family, especially the mother, needed support as they anticipated major heart surgery for Andy. The whole family could only get together on Sunday afternoons to meet with us.

On a snowy, forlorn Sunday, I drove out in the country to meet Janice at their home in one of the poorest rural areas in Illinois. After leaving the highway, I encountered barren fields—no evidence of any crops—and a cluster of rundown clapboard houses with junk cars and old door-less appliances in the yards.

Janice and I sat at the kitchen table with Dorothy, a slight dark-haired woman with no facial expression. She stared silently at the table. Susie and Andy joined us, but spookily slid on and off their chairs. Tom swaggered into the room, a big red-faced man wearing a red-plaid flannel shirt. "I'll tell you anything you want to know," he boomed. Clearly, he controlled this household.

As I set up my tape recorder in the middle of the table, I looked over Dorothy's slumped shoulders and saw something bubbling in a large aluminum pot on the old white stove. As I stared, I sensed scattered movement across the top of the stove. "Oh," I stammered, "there's something moving on your stove."

I expected them to jump up and swat dead whatever it was.

"Those are just cockroaches." Tom laughed. "The house is full of 'em. They get behind the walls, make babies, and you never get rid of 'em. Got hundreds of 'em, maybe even thousands. They're all over."

Instinctively, I lifted my feet off the floor and placed them on the chair rung. I'd seen cockroaches only once—in the basement when I was a child—and then my mother had called the exterminator right away. Even with my feet up, I imagined cockroaches scurrying up my legs. I couldn't wait to leave.

"The cats eat 'em." Tom leaned back dangerously on his chair. Yes, indeed,

I was becoming aware of more movement—this time along the floor and slithering around my legs. Black, gray, yellow—where were all the scraggily-looking cats coming from? And then I saw dogs—two big dogs with cheerless eyes, crusted noses, and clotted hair. I counted nine cats. Where were all their excretions? Suddenly, I realized the room smelled of stinky stains and hidden piles. I'd been too overwhelmed with the people to notice.

I glanced at Janice, who seemed nonplussed with the cockroaches. Stifling my horror, I said, "We're wondering what you'd like to get out of our time together."

"What do you mean?" Tom said.

"What goals do you have? As you see your situation today, what would you like to see different in the future?"

"Still don't get it," Tom said. Dorothy kept her eyes glued to the table. The kids, thin and wearing ill-fitting, mismatched clothes, retained their blank look.

"Like a one-year or five-year plan. Where would you like to be?"

"Ain't got no plans, ma'am. Just wanta have food for supper."

So Janice and I changed our focus to the absolute here-and-now needs of the family and let slide the textbook methods we were supposed to follow. We got the most valuable information from the kids, when they could slip in a word. They told us about their large extended family dropping in at any hour without knocking. Of finding an uncle in the morning sleeping off a hangover on the kitchen table. Of never knowing who'd be coming into their room. The way they talked of people coming and going in their lives felt like the way I was experiencing their helter-skelter pets and cockroaches.

Only once were Janice and I alone with the children—a split second when both parents left the room. Susie quickly slid out of her chair, stood next to my arm, and whispered directly into my ear, "My dad pees on my face when he's drunk." She added, "And he hits Mommy sometimes."

I was horrified; what else went on in this house? We reported it to our preceptor, who said incest and violence were common in these types of homes and she, as their case manager, would follow up. No consolation for me. Marianna had told me of homes she'd been in during public health nursing experiences, but I'd only half believed her until now.

Over the few Sundays that Janice and I met with this family, Dorothy brightened; she managed a washed-out smile and mumbled a few words, but I didn't feel we were making any difference. Our sessions ended with our course.

A few months later our preceptor called to say Andy was scheduled for his

surgery at a medical center in the city near our university. I visited one day after
class. After I knocked and walked into the pediatric semi-private room, Tom,
Dorothy, and Andy lit up, smiled, and hugged me. They looked strange to me
in this clean environment.

When a nurse entered the room, Dorothy exclaimed, "This is Lois. She and
Janice were our nurses at home. They helped us get ready for Andy's operation."

Perhaps we had been of help! As I left, Dorothy said, "Glad you came. We're
going to be okay here."

But I wasn't sure. I hoped she was telling the truth. I worried that abuse was
still going on in that home. I wondered if I could've done more. However, I did
sense, in their positive response, the power of our simply being there for them at
a time of extra need. I flagged in my mind that it's not necessarily just what we
say to people, but how we act: how we listen, how we encourage, how we
empathize, and how we show respect. The same lesson I'd learned as an undergraduate student three years earlier with Jenny Hart amidst the aroma of pink
roses and burnt toast.

By spring quarter of the first year, Marianna and I were surprised to find we could
take one course together. Her specialty required a health assessment course; mine
did not, but since my federal grant did, we arranged to take this course at the same
time. In this class, we were taught how to take patient histories and to perform
physical exams. Marianna and I, of course, chose each other as lab partners.

What we learned encompassed much more than we'd ever experienced in
any doctor's office. We asked every possible question for the history, and we
probed every possible body part for the physical. Well, not quite. We were spared
the pelvic and rectal exams. But no history of hernias, heartburn, hemorrhoids,
or heat intolerance escaped us. And, after the physical, nothing was sacred—not
our lumps, rashes, thyroids, livers, heart sounds, lung sounds, peripheral pulses,
or peristaltic waves rippling across the abdomen. Not even breasts. And this presented me with more of a problem, I think, than Marianna. In this area, she was
more than twice my size, and, sure, we knew each other well, but not this well.
I methodically demonstrated my new, round-the-clock palpation techniques—
kneading and lifting each breast as if it were a loaf of bread dough. Luckily, Marianna kept her eyes on the ceiling. When it was her turn to examine me, she was
done in a snap. Not as much dough. At the completion of this course, we knew

more about each other than our husbands knew—or would care to know. And it had been great fun being able to study together, to quiz each other on the hundreds of terms used in the review of body systems and on the sequence of the 101 steps of the final exam. For the exam, we had to bring in our own patient. Another classmate volunteered her husband for me. The instructor sat at the foot of the bed in the nursing lab with a checklist of the 101 items we had to cover. My "patient" had a "bump" on his left ear that I couldn't figure out how to describe—the right term escaped me—and afterward, I chided my classmate for not warning me.

When we passed this exam, which took us each two hours, Marianna and I were exuberant. We had the knowledge and potential to be more thorough than any doctor's physical we'd ever had. We were indeed getting quantifiably smarter.

In my final clinical course, consultation-liaison nursing, I learned how to be a resource for staff, patients, and families. For their educational and emotional needs. As a former med-surg nurse, I chose to do this clinical on an oncology unit. In my earlier staff nursing days, oncology units didn't exist, but I'd had many patients diagnosed with cancer on my wards.

My preceptor, a nurse with a master's degree in psychiatric nursing (the unit's clinical nurse specialist—CNS), addressed both educational and emotional needs of all the people on her unit. I followed her on her rounds of mostly terminally ill patients who lay weakened in their beds. This was before there was much success with radiation or chemotherapy treatments. She'd sit close to the patient at eye level, smile, talk softly, listen, pat their hands, and finish by saying, "See you tomorrow. You know you can call for me anytime." She offered a breath of hope.

When we got out into the hallway between patients, she'd say, "Okay, Lois. Stand up straight. Roll your shoulders back, take a deep breath, and smile. Let go of that patient, so you'll be fresh for the next one." Advice I tried to follow the rest of my career.

After every death on the unit, the preceptor convened a staff meeting and took me along to observe. "How are you going to handle this one?" She expected each person to respond. One new grandma said, "I'm stopping at my daughter's after work to hold my new grandbaby. I need to know that life goes on." Others spoke of going to a movie or to the gym to work out. I could not fathom dealing with constant deaths on the unit as well as these people did.

The preceptor also directed me to sit in the floor's solarium, a sunny room at the end of the hall, with family members who came in and out for a breather from the intensity of sitting at the bedside of their loved ones. "Here are people who also need our help. Do your thing. Listen."

I didn't guess then that I'd be one of these family members later in life. These people, eager to be heard, told dozens of painful stories: aloof doctors, mouth sores from medication, and relatives not dying at the projected time. One older woman in the solarium said, "I can't cry anymore. He was supposed to die six weeks ago. Even he feels like he's a burden to us now. We're just biding time and spending up our savings. He's worried about how I'll get along after he finally goes."

After she left, I stopped in to see her husband. He corroborated her story. "They should never tell you it's going to be six months. Because then you plan on six months. And it's a shame if you don't meet the deadline. I feel like everyone's just waiting for me to go." He stared out the window, maybe sensing that I didn't know any words to say that could comfort him. But I did know how to listen, to show him someone cared enough to simply sit there. The desolate sound of his voice describing "not meeting the deadline" haunts me yet today when I listen to a friend or family member express similar feelings during their final days.

After two years as a full-time student, the excitement of learning, conducting research, and hobnobbing the city with Marianna on our sanity breaks came to an end. For a final breakfast, we went to Lou Mitchell's, southwest of the Loop at Jackson and Clinton, and shared one of their famous frying pan omelets. We did not share their complementary Milk Duds, though. Coming for an early lunch after classes, we had closed this place down at its closing time of 3:00 many times. We talked about "now what?" We were headed back to our respective suburbs—an hour apart, back to being more available wives and moms, and back to thinking about work. We made plans to meet in the Loop at least once a month. We talked maybe of doing the next degree together—a doctorate—but only after our kids were off to college, at least five years away.

Boarding the Illinois Central train for my last trip home, I pressed "Play" and "Record" on my bulky black Panasonic tape recorder—no such thing yet as a microcassette—stashed in my backpack. I taped the sounds of the train and the conductor calling out station stops. When longings for the city seeped into my suburban consciousness, I could play my very own train song: clickety-clack…115ᵗʰ and Kensington…clickety-clack…Riverdale…clickety-clack…Olympia Fields…clickety-clack…Matteson.

After I got off the train, I walked south on Main, dipped under the viaduct, and headed toward 218ᵗʰ Street—the short, curved, cut-through street to the open field behind our home on Winnebago. As I rounded the corner on 218ᵗʰ, I spotted Kathleen at the end of the block. A tall sixth-grader now, she spotted me and started running toward me, waving. We met mid-block and hugged, a ritual we'd had on my school days. "We just got home from the orthodontist and now Dad's making supper." She smiled, huffing. "He's making lasagna, our favorite frozen On-Cor stuff." It would be good to be home more, to have a reprieve from studying, and to be more available for my family. While I'd been on the graduate school train runs, Jon and Kath had grown taller than I, and their teeth had gotten straighter, thanks to Marv's many trips to the orthodontist. In the acknowledgment to my master's thesis, I wrote: "A special thank you goes to my family. Jon, my fourteen-year-old son, humored me often by telling me I could be doing two theses instead of one. Kathleen, my eleven-year-old daughter, studied quietly with me for many hours and kept us well supplied with candy and beverages. Marv, my husband and partner, unselfishly held our household together and gave me boundless emotional support."

As Kathleen and I, hand in hand, skipped across the open field toward our back yard, I saw the leaves on Marv's dwarf apple trees gently moving in the warm wind. I imagined they were waving a welcome home. I glanced up at the clear blue sky and whispered a prayer of thanks.

Twelve

CLEANING HOUSE

*W*e have state-of-the-art equipment to recover our ECT patients in this room." The head nurse beamed as she talked. I folded my bare arms to try to keep warm as I recalled my morning shifts as a teenager in the late fifties working switchboard at Pine Rest. While I said, "Good morning, Pine Rest," patients from the women's ward behind my cubicle would be coming back from their electroconvulsive therapy treatments. I would cringe as I heard moaning and be tempted to open the back door of my space to peek.

As I stood looking at the lineup of empty beds made up with crisp white linens, I recalled one of my master's professors telling us about her experiences in the late seventies with unsuccessful ECT treatment. The negatives in my mind shadowed my mood even though I'd learned that ECT was greatly changed and now successful. I shivered in the chill of the shiny steel and glass recovery room. I'd not worn a sweater for this late summer interview for the clinical nurse specialist position at a new one-hundred-bed psychiatric hospital. It'd been a few months since I'd graduated, and I was itchy to see what kind of jobs I would qualify for with my new master's.

After the tour of the psych units and the ECT suite, the head nurse led me back to her office. "I'd like to offer you the position."

I was shocked. The offer came too easily, reminding me of the teaching offer I'd received on my first interview after I'd finished my bachelor's. Driving home, I felt like an imposter—a med-surg nurse parading as a psych nurse just because I now had a master's in the field. Was this what I wanted to do? Me, who liked the faster-paced busyness of med-surg units? Would I even like this head-more-than-body type of nursing?

The job's hours were 7:00 to 4:00. Now that I was finished with school, I'd told Marv I would get the kids off to school. Since the starting time was too early, I had to turn down the position. I would later regret I'd not had hands-on experience on a psychiatric unit.

My second interview was at a general hospital. I was offered the position as the coordinator of nursing education. This hospital was closer to home and the hours were 8:00 to 4:00. The coordinator oversaw employee orientations and in-service programs ranging from CPR renewals to medical terminology classes to new product information. The range of programs sounded like a good way to keep current. I accepted the offer, and since it was my first street clothes desk job, I saw it as an opportunity to buy my first Evan Picone suit—gray flannel with a sewed-down pleated skirt.

The first day, after one hour of reading policy manuals, my staff of three RNs rescued me to go for coffee. We walked two city blocks of hallways to the hospital cafeteria with its shelves of fresh frosted donuts and sweet rolls. At first glance across the cafeteria, it looked as if quite a few staff had consumed these pastries for years. We trekked back to the cafeteria at noon and at three for coffee again. Both times, I noted the calorie-heavy desserts and heavy people waddling down the hall for more. At four, I went home.

I thought back to a master's class in which we had read Erving Goffman's *Asylums* and learned that patients, upon a lengthy hospitalization, would assume characteristics of the institution. I thought, *how true, and it doesn't have to be a psychiatric stay*. It appeared that employees, after many treks to the cafeteria, could exemplify the types of food they'd eaten. Were the jobs here so unfulfilling that the joy was in the sweets? I asked my staff not to get me for coffee twice a day anymore. Besides, I thought, what a waste of time traveling hallways—about fifteen minutes each way.

After only a few days, the director of nursing called me in and informed me that my department's staff and educational programs had been status quo for a long while. "I'd like you to conduct a needs assessment and see if your department can meet the educational needs you identify."

I had not been told of the "status quo" in my initial interview with the director of education; I felt set up to clean house.

After gathering my staff to tell them what we'd been commanded to do, I conducted the assessment, drawing on research skills I had learned doing my master's thesis, and, of course, major changes had to be made. For starters, none of the staff had advanced knowledge and skills in coronary or intensive care. In fact, other than the director of nursing and her assistant, I was only the third nurse at the hospital who held a master's degree.

As the results rolled in from the needs assessment, the staff members knew their time was limited. One pragmatically found another job; another successfully designed a position for herself in a different hospital department; and the final one graciously accepted returning to the floor as a night nurse—work she felt too old to do, but had no choice financially. When she left, she told me, "I'd love to hate you for this, Lois, but I find I can't."

It did not feel good to edge these people out of their jobs, and I admired the women for dealing with the demise of their long-held positions so well. I also admired them for not sending me to the lion's den when I forbade smoking in one office held by two of the women. Years of paperwork had yellowed on the shelves from the smoke.

I was the only one to leave the department totally voluntarily. As I reflected on my leaving—I had no interest in setting up a new department—I also thought back to why I'd taken this job. My former advisor in the bachelor's program, the one who pushed for my education minor, had called me about the position. She held it at the time and was leaving it for a nursing administration job in the same hospital. But when I took the job, she never talked to me. Once, at lunchtime, I approached her table of administrative people in the cafeteria and asked if I could join them. She replied, without her former teacher smile, "No, we're having a meeting." Never once did she call me or visit me in her old office. Not having the guts to confront her, I surmised she knew she had set me up to be a hatchet woman and couldn't or didn't want to face me.

She left behind a crucifix, hanging on the soffit above her desk. It had apparently fallen at one time because its legs were broken. From my view seated below it, the shins lunged toward me, while the jagged thighs pointed aimlessly beyond my back. It looked as if it needed knees to hold them together.

Not being Catholic, having a crucifix hanging above my head was a new experience. Its brokenness struck me as oddly funny. Wasn't it sacrilegious not to replace it with a whole one? I told my family that the job wasn't going as well as I had hoped, but neither had the God hanging above my head fared very well. In Dutch, my mother had a word for my humor: *spotten* (to mock). On the other hand, never having had a religious icon, the symbol of Christ's presence watching over me, in spite of fractured legs, gave me a warmed sense of peace in a situation of alienation.

As my staff was leaving, I interviewed for a new patient education position being developed at the hospital. The administrator with whom I met said, "Lois, I know you wouldn't be happy in this position. Teaching patients wouldn't keep you stimulated. You belong with professionals."

I was furious. What did he know about me? More than I gave him credit for at the time.

So I interviewed for a faculty position back at Prairie State College, the community college where I'd started my teaching career. The academic vice-president asked, "Why are you coming back? Why are you taking a $10,000 pay cut?" The job offered $17,000 for a nine-month contract, compared to the $27,000 a year I was making.

I said, "I'd rather work with people than paper."

During my final weeks, I picked up teaching the classes my former staff had run for years: medical terminology to unit secretaries and diabetic teaching to patients. I enjoyed these few hours each week. Relearning prefixes, root words, and suffixes for medical terms was a good review for me. Even though I had never taught a theory class and had no idea how to teach the subject, I muddled through, trying to keep in mind that I knew more than the students. And I loved the patient contact in the class for patients with diabetes. One man stayed afterwards to tell me of his problem with impotence. "I've never told anyone before." We sat across from each other at a narrow conference table and he poured out his story of years of grief and shame. He had never shared his problem with his internist, and the internist had never asked. My tears welled up as I felt his pain. That he entrusted me with his story felt overwhelming. I was happy I could help him by listening and by guiding him to a urology referral.

The rest of each week, I spent hours alone in my old musty basement office administering the tuition reimbursement program. Early on, the director of the department had resigned, so his responsibilities of the past year, including the reimbursement program, had fallen to me. In between the boring paperwork, I interviewed for my replacement. One who would start a new staff education department from scratch. In my appointment book, the first I'd ever needed, I crossed off the days until I could leave.

Thirteen

LIVERWURST

he spiral chrome neck of the portable microphone swung its head away from me in defiance. "Stop it," I muttered. "Stop wiggling!" I was practicing for my first major lecture ever. A lecture I would give to 100 brand-new nursing students. The teaching podium, a long laboratory desk with Bunsen burners at both ends, smelled like the sulphuric acid of my college chemistry lab in 1959.

Back at my desk that fall of 1982, I stared at ten pages of handwritten notes, trying to memorize parts at the last minute, not seeing a single word. Hands planted themselves on my shoulders. I knew it could only be Maureen, my former psychiatric nursing mentor. She would be retiring soon, and I would replace her. Kneading the stress knots in my neck, she chanted, "You can do this, you can do this. Remember, they don't know you've never done this before. Remember, you know more than they do. Remember to bluff it."

Her words formed a mantra in my mind.

I carried my new cowhide briefcase into the deep rectangular lecture room. Staring at the rows of faces—a mixed group of age, gender, and ethnicity, but mostly white females—I did not know if the lecture I'd written would last thirty minutes or three hours, or if I'd be able to maintain order if the class did not pay attention.

Sitting in armchair desks, the students stared back at me. One immediate attention problem sat near the back row, miles away, on the left side of the middle aisle. I figured out his name from my class list, called on him, and cracked a joke—the first of many to pop from a previously unknown joke box in my brain. I was on a high, off and running.

I had too many notes for fifty minutes. This was better, though, than running short. I feared even thirty seconds with nothing to say and the wild horseplay I was certain would ensue. Probably because that was me as a student—on the lookout for fun.

For that first class, I wore my new teaching clothes—sage pull-on slacks, peach ruffled blouse, and dark green belted cardigan. I handled the microphone. I held attention. I taught the class. Strutting back to my office, I felt as if I'd found a stage of my own.

Before school had started, I'd met with my three team teachers of the nursing foundations course to divvy up the teaching load. I worried I'd get the leftovers, what the others didn't want. I hated the heart—I never wanted to learn the blood vessel stuff again—and I loathed the lungs, especially mucus spewing forth from tracheotomies. I was assigned the gastrointestinal system, mouth to anus, under modules titled Nutrition and Elimination. Fortunately for me, the others hated these topics. In contrast to my early med-surg days, I no longer minded emptying bedpans. In fact, I felt what my friends called a "perverse pleasure" when the full bedpan I was carrying had made my patient feel better.

"Today, we're starting the elimination module," I announced mid-semester to the array of faces resembling a field of sunflowers. "First, we need to know how food is propelled by a series of reflexes through the digestive tract to the end of its journey. This will explain why we need to toilet our nursing home patients soon after breakfast.

"Let's take a patient example, Janie." I pointed to a middle-aged woman sitting in a front row seat on my left. "Let's think of your patient Mr. Kline at Cherry Creek Care Center. First, you wheeled Mr. Kline down to the dining room to eat his breakfast. The food—French toast and orange juice—traveled down his esophagus to the stomach. There, the gastrocolic reflex propelled it forward into the small intestine. Then the duodenocolic reflex propelled it to the large intestine."

I sneaked my hands under the lab desk to get a cellophane-wrapped tube of liverwurst wrapped in red yarn. Whipping it up to the level of my chin, I said, "This is like the large intestine. About two inches in diameter, in contrast to the one inch of the small intestine, and the red yarn symbolizes the mesenteric artery that nourishes the colon. And we have one more reflex to go: the defecation reflex that causes release of the bowel movement."

Unobtrusively, I pricked the tube with a safety pin and began to squeeze it high above the desk. A thin paste of liverwurst wound its way down to my eye level where it began to break off in ribbons that fell, kerplop, on the desk. Students stared in shock. Then waves of giggles burst around the room.

Later, in shopping malls, I would meet graduates who'd remind me they were from the "liverwurst class," as if membership earned them a badge of humor. At least they remembered my lecture! One said, "I haven't eaten liverwurst since."

Fourteen

OSCAR MAYER WEINER

*S*tanding barefoot on our brown tweed kitchen carpeting, I leaned against the orange Formica bar to steady myself against feelings of shock, excitement, and fright. Had I heard right?

I'd been reading, flopped on a blue print velour couch (part of a new four-piece set from Wickes) in the living room, when the phone had rung at 10:30. Marv and the kids were long in bed. I'd scrambled to the kitchen to answer the wall phone by the back door. The caller introduced herself as the director of the new nursing department at Trinity Christian College, seventeen miles northwest from us. "I got your name as someone who may be interested in coming to help us start a baccalaureate nursing program. We need a person with a psychiatric nursing master's who can also teach foundations."

My exact qualifications. But why such a late call? Desperate? Me, the gal who may have a diploma mentality forever. Would I even be able to teach baccalaureate students? Plus it was June already, and I had already signed my 1983-84 contract.

"Go for it, Lois," my Prairie State chairperson said. "As you said, the college has your Dutch background…your Christian Reformed church background, plus it's an opportunity to teach baccalaureate."

After my interviews with nursing faculty, college faculty, the academic dean, the college president, and board of trustees' representatives, Marv and I decided I would accept the position. Along with psychiatric nursing, I could still teach nutrition and elimination, the GI system, that I now liked. And, after hours of family discussion, Marv, Jon, Kathleen and I decided, even though I could commute, we would move closer to the college. It would be about the same distance for Marv to go to work, and then Jon, as a junior, and Kathleen, as a freshman, could attend a Christian high school with the same faith as our church. Many of their cousins attended a Christian school, as had Marv and I, and they were curious how it might differ from their public school.

But moving to this new community for my job totally disrupted our kids' lives. They were used to having good friends and not having to crack into strongly formed cliques to find new friends. Roller coaster moods careened through the house every evening. I listened, hour after hour, and also had to do hours of work. Many nights, after Marv and the kids were asleep, I locked myself in the bathroom, doubled over in painful silent tears, and prayed, *Please, God, help make it possible for us to move back to Park Forest.* Our former home hadn't sold. We'd tripled our mortgage payment and assumed thousands of dollars in tuition. For what?

Having relocated primarily for the kids' school, it seemed like a long time before all of us could appreciate the move. We even gave the kids' the choice to transfer to the local public high school, which they refused, not knowing what they would encounter there. I was grateful to one of my colleagues at Trinity who said to me one day while eating lunch at a picnic table in the quad, "Lois, my daughter is one of the many kids at the school who can't accept new kids like yours. They're all Dutch, they've all gone to school together since kindergarten, and many are interrelated. My daughter and her friends are so insecure that they don't make a move without checking with each other." So at least I could tell my kids to not take the ostracism personally, that maybe it was more the other kids' problems than theirs.

At the start of my second year, our department secretary came to the nursing lab on a Tuesday in September while I was doing return demonstrations of bedpan placement with the students. She called me out from behind the curtain. "The dean would like to see you when you're finished."

Now what? I had no idea. I completed supervising the students and scurried the short distance to the dean's office. He said our director would be leaving and asked if I would assume "acting director" starting Thursday. He said he'd checked with the other nursing faculty, and they were willing to work with me.

I wasn't aware any of those discussions had been taking place. Did I have a choice?

A memo came out on September 25, 1984: "Mrs. Lois Roelofs has been named acting director until a permanent replacement can be secured."

I had two days of orientation to the file cabinets in the director's office. The mail, phone calls, and department problems guided the rest of my orientation that year. Having only an observer's knowledge of what a director did in a baccalaureate program, or any kind of program, I learned on the job, minute by minute, by what came across my desk. I tried to be proactive, ferreting out and addressing potential problems before they could occur.

I soon realized running a nursing program was not unlike my experience as a head nurse, only now I was running a department with faculty and students instead of a ward with staff and patients. At least no one was sick here. The major CPR I would perform would be on the paperwork of the program. And though the paperwork was not sick, per se, keeping it up to snuff required constant attention. Because we were a new program, we needed to get our completed set of syllabi approved by the state. The academic dean and I traveled to the capitol to meet with the nurse examining board. We sat on one side of a large square of tables. The members flanked the other three sides. While pushing our stack of syllabi away from her, one member turned her entire body to the side and informed the group she had never seen such a lack of consistency in course content. She used a less constructive expression, and there was no way I could miss her point. Another person pointed out that our syllabi didn't specify that we gave our students a lunch break during clinical time, so did that mean we didn't actually have the required number of clinical hours that we were supposed to have or did it mean that we were not going to allow our students to eat? It was not the climate to show amusement, so I made a note to be sure to feed our students and document those details in the future.

After this informative session of how *not* to mentor or encourage lesser-experienced faculty like me, the dean and I decided to hire a consultant to help us tighten our curriculum. The course content was sound, but we, the small faculty covering adult, maternal and child, community health, and mental health nursing, needed guidance to show how we made the roles of the nurse—caregiver, communicator, researcher, and teacher—consistent and clear to the students throughout each course. We worked dozens of hours, including over Christmas break. We didn't get Christmas cookies made or presents wrapped, but we did master the tree branch structure—formally called the threads and strands—of curriculum development. We became curriculum experts and kept up our morale with lots of joking. As we floundered writing dozens of learning objectives, we'd laugh, parroting out loud the repetitious phrases, probably not realizing at the time that each of us could, at the completion of our work, verbally recite, word for word, all the objectives of the program and of all the courses, totaling fifty-five credit hours.

Sometimes CPR was necessary on the students' parents. When we as faculty planned a multiethnic community health experience in the city of Chicago, a parent called demanding to know if we were aware that the agency we had chosen was placed at the most unsafe five-corner intersection in the city. Along with the college president and the academic dean, we quickly called a parent informational meeting. Words flew concerning student safety until one parent stood up and said he worked in the area and most of the corner's inhabitants would still be dead drunk asleep on the street in the early morning when our students got there. So no real threat. And we had to reassure the parents that our program accreditation guidelines required exposure to diverse situations. And we had to point out to them that even though they sent their children to our small Christian college in the suburbs thinking they would be safe there, nursing was not limited to caring for people in cloistered environments. That first class of twenty-one students seemed to thrive on the city experience. It almost felt like they were out to show their parents they could and wanted to become city savvy. For all, it was their first extended experience, if not first trip, into that area of Chicago. When I asked once what was the most fun thing they learned, several giggled and said, "To parallel park." Coming from small towns or suburbs, they'd never had to sandwich their car into a small space on a busy city street. Two even admitted a cop had approached them as they walked along a deserted street and told them they didn't belong there, it wasn't safe. "Don't let anyone know we did this," they begged me. "We won't do it again."

That spring, managing to survive the paperwork and parental challenges, I was a total failure teaching the mental health nursing course for the first time. I had no time to prepare. And that was when I became acutely aware I'd never had staff experience on a psych unit. I had my degree that gave me theoretical knowledge, but my clinical knowledge was limited to my own student experiences and those as a clinical instructor. To survive teaching the course, I divvied up the modules into student presentations. They hated doing them. They saw through my ruse.

I never did that again. And I'm thankful to those first graduates of our program for not staging an uprising in my course. I strongly sensed one student's ire, though, with my delegation method. I felt for her; she reminded me a lot of myself as a student. And I thought it ironic at graduation when we both showed up in the same style dress, different colors.

By the fall of 1986, my third year, our search for a new director holding a doctorate had been successful and I was back in the classroom and clinical where I wanted to be. Back to the challenges of adapting my teaching style from what worked with my older community college students to my current younger four-year college students. I fearlessly had taken this position. After my previous success at Prairie State, and despite the mental health nursing course the spring before, I expected to be dynamite. After being accustomed to a class of 100 in a room the size of a banquet hall, a class of twenty at Trinity seemed like a small family dinner.

Once, in a lecture course on foundational concepts in nursing, I taught in a square classroom holding six round tables surrounded by young, mostly blonde, females. From the start, entire tables of students would giggle, smirk, or frown when least expected. I figured out that those with their backs to me were making faces I couldn't see. What was wrong? How could this happen? How would I deal with it? This certainly didn't feel like a cozy family dinner. I felt more like the oddball Aunt Bertha nobody had wanted to invite.

I never thought to rearrange the room.

The jokes that worked at Prairie State didn't work here. Sullen stares froze my humor midair. It was as if I had to prove something to win them over. But what? I swear the students schemed to not smile at my jokes. They succeeded.

In a desperate attempt to get a reaction, any reaction, during a communication lecture about Eric Berne's transactional analysis theory, I remembered a skit I had performed at Governors State University in the middle seventies while getting my bachelor's degree. My class had been instructed to demonstrate Berne's child, adult, and parent modes of communication. My subgroup quickly cooked up a skit in the playful mode of Berne's "spontaneous child." Squatting on each other's backs, we formed a human pyramid, cocked our heads up toward our classmates, and droned the Oscar Mayer wiener song. Our classmates had roared.

Now, I pulled up my narrow, calf-length, charcoal-gray skirt so I could get down on the floor. On my hands and knees, I sang the song with all the fervor of a hotdog wanting to be loved.

Students peered around each other's heads to glimpse me wailing country-music style on the floor, all forty-three years of me acting as childish as I could possibly get—as desperate as I was willing to act. They shielded their mouths with their hands, snickered, and whispered. No audible reaction. Didn't they know they were acting out the "adapted child" of Berne's theory? The ones who behaved as they'd been programmed to do? Couldn't they let go and find their "spontaneous child"?

I rose to my feet, dismissed the class. In silence, they filed out until they reached the hallway. There, I heard rumbles of chatter.

I wanted to stomp out the door after them and scream, "What's the matter, guys? I like fun, don't you like fun? I know this is heavy stuff to learn, but can't you lighten up a bit?"

But I didn't confront them. I moped. I wished my Maureen from Prairie State would show up and massage my shoulders. I had no mentor here. I was alone on the stage. I, as an actress, wasn't having fun.

And my audience wasn't either, so almost every day required soul searching. If a teaching approach hadn't worked, I had to try something new. I don't remember making any conscious choice to change, but do remember thinking I would have to get back the confidence I'd gained at Prairie State and start trusting who I was again.

One day in a nursing home clinical, while shaking down a glass thermometer to below 98.6, a student dropped it on a tiled floor. I found her mortified under the bed trying to gather up splinters of glass with a tissue. With my elbows and hips, I scooted under the bed on my stomach, head low, with wet paper towel in hand to chase the beads of mercury that eluded our pursuit and shot ahead of us to the other side of the bed. We had to giggle and hoped we didn't further confuse the already confused patient lying above us. We didn't know at that time that we shouldn't be trying to catch mercury by hand. After emerging from under that bed, it became easier and easier to become my silly self.

After supper on our evening shifts in a Christian nursing home, we held hymn sings because, as a child, I had loved playing and singing hymns. I was always blessed with a student who could play the piano, so I could lead the singing. Students were surprised that patients, not even knowing their own names, could sing all the verses of old favorites. "Amazing Grace." "On the Old Rugged Cross." "What a Friend We Have in Jesus."

Trying to introduce some humor into the mental health nursing lectures, when we were studying what foods not to eat with certain psychiatric meds, I brought a platter full of the offenders from my kitchen into class for the students to memorize. I told them when they got a test question about them, all they'd have to do was visualize the plate: banana, aged cheese, chocolate, wine.... The platter evoked a lot of chatter and laughs.

Still, I was thrilled in 1987 when the college granted my request for an unpaid one-year leave to return for my doctorate. Once again, I would be able to do my favorite things: wear jeans, crew neck sweaters, tennis shoes. Carry a backpack. Bum around with fellow students. Crack new books. Prowl library stacks. Hear lectures instead of give them. Learn.

Kathleen would start Calvin College that fall and Jon would be a junior. Because I had worked full-time the previous year, we didn't qualify for financial aid. To everyone he met, Marv good-naturedly said, "I'm going to have to start bagging groceries at night. I have to support three kids in college next year." And Trinity even graciously arranged a salary schedule that would pay me half time for the next two years to give me some income during the year I was on leave.

I was blessed.

PART FOUR

Doctorate

Fifteen

COGITO ERGO SUM

here'd the time go?" I asked Marv as we drove in the early autumn afternoon sun from Grand Rapids toward Saugatuck. "I can't believe it's over. It seems like yesterday that I couldn't get pregnant. And now the kids are both gone."

"Yeah," he said, "it feels good."

That day we had settled Kathleen into her dorm room at Calvin College. Not at the Franklin Street campus, the old one-block-square site dating back to 1917, where we had met twenty-eight years earlier. But the Knollcrest campus built on the edge of town on wooded land first purchased in 1956. We'd had our freshman mixer there—a picnic with hot dogs and rope pullings. As we'd carried Kath's jeans, linens, and typewriter into her dorm and meandered around the sprawling campus, over 300 acres of hilly, tree-filled land, I looked around wistfully. I tried to feel connected. I couldn't. The setting was strange, and in our strongly intertwined Dutch community, I was surprised I didn't run into any parents I knew.

That day, September 8, 1987, was our twenty-fifth anniversary. We were officially empty nesters. Jon had driven himself to Calvin and was already settled in for his junior year.

And, at age forty-five, I would soon be on my way to becoming a full-time student again at the University of Illinois. To get a head start, I'd taken two seminar courses during the summer.

I had wanted to return for the PhD since I'd left with my master's in 1981. In fact, at that time, I'd been envious of the one student in my class who'd stayed on to do the master's bypass program to complete the PhD. With my kids only eleven and thirteen at the time, I was torn between my children's need for having me available during their teen years and my love of learning and desire for a doctorate. The kids, of course, won out. The doctorate was postponed. For Marianna, too, for the same reasons.

For over a year, I had prepared for my academic leave. I studied again for the Graduate Record Exam. For the verbal part, I learned 1,000 vocabulary words, carrying old flash cards from Marv's Calvin days everywhere I went. On a trip from Chicago to Seattle with my older nurse-sister Kay, who was starting a dean position, I quizzed her through the national parks: Badlands, Grand Teton, Yellowstone, and Glacier. On a vacation to Long Island in which Marv and I took my folks back for a celebration at one of my dad's former churches, the four of us quizzed each other as we traveled through Ohio, Pennsylvania, and New York. The only word I remember now is "ubiquitous," which describes the state of my study materials as I updated myself for taking the GREs.

For the math section, I met Marianna in the city to take a ten-week review course at the University of Illinois. The teacher must've known how hopeless some of us were, because he told us what type of problems to skip. Blank answers wouldn't count against us, while wrong answers would. For the analytical part of the test, Marianna and I worked numerous problems from a GRE study book.

I was worried, having been the oldest in my master's class, that I surely would be one of the oldest students in the doctoral class. Nurses, historically, had raised children first and earned advanced degrees later. And if they got doctorates, those degrees were often earned in areas such as education, psychology, or physiology, because doctoral programs in nursing were not available.

The University of Illinois started the first PhD program in nursing in the seventies. By 1987, when I was starting, the PhD in nursing was considered the crème de la crème of degrees. The rumor among nurses was, "If you're younger than fifty, the terminal degree—the doctorate—must be in nursing; if older than fifty, it doesn't matter." My sister Kay had gotten her doctorate in counseling psychology, and, even though I'd explored that doctorate and others in psychology, she strongly urged me to get mine in nursing.

And, by 1987, younger nurses were pursuing advanced degrees. Would I feel rusty next to students half my age? I wanted to be able to hold my own among them. I didn't want them to know, for example, that before I'd taken the math review course, I hadn't known that an integer is a whole number. I felt dated in the simplest of things.

Also, would I be able to withstand the rigor of the coursework and then the dissertation? As much as I'd wanted to do this and had looked forward to it, suddenly I thought the idea might be preposterous. I'd gotten tired in my teaching life, and I had no assurance that I could sail through a student life, along with a commute, and still have time awake to spend with Marv.

And I was sad that Marianna and I would not be getting this degree together. Since taking the math review course, Marianna had rethought getting a doctorate. As a nurse practitioner, her job didn't require one, and she loved the direct patient contact. She was a loyal friend who had made getting our bachelor's and master's fun. I would miss her terribly.

To celebrate our twenty-fifth anniversary, Marv and I stayed overnight in Saugatuck, a quaint town with rustic shops. We climbed the 900 steps of Mt. Baldy and, afterwards, reminisced over ice cream cones about our camping days with the kids at nearby Goshorn Lake when they were little.

When we got home, there were a few weeks before my doctoral program started. I found myself in a silent house running on automatic. When I heard a neighbor teen call "mom" outside, I darted to the front door. When I drove past the high school tennis courts, I looked over to see if Kath was there among the tall blondes in their purple and gold uniforms. When I made lunch, I checked the clock to make sure the time coincided with Jon's lunch hour from the lumberyard. With each incident, it dawned on me the kids were gone and I was truly empty nested and about to start on another road of my career.

My first day finally came. Driving north in my orange '83 Renault Alliance on the Stevenson Expressway (there was no convenient train from Palos Heights), I exited left on Damen while listening to Patsy Cline's "One Day at a Time, Sweet Jesus."

Ever cheap, I parked free on Roosevelt Road next to abandoned buildings in the process of urban renewal, walked three blocks up, and settled into a tenth floor graduate student office in the psychiatric nursing department. I felt as if I'd never left. I looked out the window facing Taylor and sensed, once again, the excitement of the crowded city.

I plunged into the three-quarter sequence of core courses in theories, research, and statistics, plus the required electives. I needed to pull brain cells out of storage to tackle the required reading, often more than 100 pages per week in each course.

I'd never had such demands on my time before. I quickly figured out I had to read for one course each night in order to make time to write papers on days I didn't have class. I instituted a system for myself that I had devised for my students. I'd suggest to them, when they were distraught from the amount of homework the nursing major required, to divide their week into twenty-one time blocks—morning, afternoon, and evening for each day. I'd show them how to draw an expanded tic tac toe grid. Then I'd tell them to X out each square where their time was committed—class, work, church. And to leave, for their mental health, one time block open each week, for play.

Sunday nights, I filled in my grid for the following week. I learned if I didn't get the reading done for each course in its slotted time block, it wouldn't get read. Having the time constraint helped me speed up my reading, but also made me a jittery wreck. Eventually, I relaxed and got a rhythm. I left Friday evenings open for Marv; they became pizza nights at Aurelio's. We settled into a booth and caught up on each other's week over pepperoni pizza and a jug of root beer. Luckily, he dashed along at a galloping pace himself, so my new schedule worked out satisfactorily for both of us.

The first course in the theories core was a Philosophy of Science course. I had never taken any course in philosophy. The first day, I deduced logic must have been prerequisite knowledge as only one class period was devoted to it. When I got home, I dug out Marv's college logic book from the attic and taught myself a three-hour course that evening. I learned about syllogisms—if every A is a C and B is an A, then B will be a C. Simple! I could understand by substituting a patient experience. If all my patients are pre-ops and Mr. Jones is my patient, then he will be a pre-op. I decided my one-night stand with logic was easier than taking a semester-long course.

But the philosophy course demanded more than logic. "You'll need to pick out a philosopher from the schedule in the syllabus and co-lead a discussion in class," the professor said. "This will constitute twenty-five percent of your grade."

I scanned the list. After an introduction to theory building during week two, we covered one philosopher per week: Aristotle, Descartes, Hume, Kant, Hempel, Popper, and Kuhn. Interesting names, but I didn't know them. Not knowing any of my new classmates either, I jumped in: "I'll work with someone on Descartes."

I pronounced both S's. Someone whispered the correct pronunciation to me.

I had three weeks to prepare, but first I had to read Dubin's 300-page *Theory Building* for the next week. To learn again, but more in-depth this time, what a theory is and what distinguishes a weak theory from a strong one. For the following week, I had to read Aristotle's *Nicomachean Ethics.* Plus I had the reading for the three other courses I was taking.

The second I got home, I called my philosophy colleague at Trinity. "Help! I need you to teach me everything I need to know about Descartes and how he fits into the philosophy of science so I can give a two-hour presentation. My schedule is tight. I can manage two hours. Will you do it?"

Having recently finished a lengthy doctorate, he laughed. I heard him call out to his colleague in the adjacent office. "Lois is on the phone. She wants to know everything there is to know about Descartes in two hours." Still chuckling, he came back on the phone. "Sure, I can teach you everything I know in two hours." He laughed again. "We can, at least, try our best to make you sound smart."

The next week, armed with a class outline of what was expected in the presentation and my copies of Descartes' *Discourse on Method* and *Meditations on First Philosophy* that I'd read and underlined, I sat with my colleague at his dining room table and concentrated hard late into the evening.

He was a good tutor. When I got an A on the presentation, I called to thank him. He hadn't accepted my offer to pay him for his help, so I sent him and his wife a floral centerpiece in browns and oranges for their fall table. I was very grateful. I never could've assimilated the knowledge in such a short time period without his clear guidance.

"Cogito ergo sum." That's about all I remember about Descartes. I still love the sound of the phrase. And I do remember it has something to do with rationalism versus empiricism. And I will stop there.

This time around, I loved the courses in my research core. Especially the first one, because of the youngish lanky male professor. He lectured slowly and distinctly. I could easily take notes. The textbook he'd chosen for the class had bold black headings and ample white space. I could grasp reading the organized material on the clean-looking pages without feeling like I was going to stroke out. His wry smiles captivated me. I wondered how my students had felt about my humor. His cute grin, when he'd refer to "recommended readings" in the library, motivated me to hustle over there to find them and read them all.

His tests, however, defied any experience I'd ever had. "There will be five essay questions," he explained. "They will test your ability to synthesize the lectures, the textbook, and all the readings on reserve in the library."

After he handed out the first test, I blanked momentarily. I was used to multiple-choice questions. On a clean sheet of paper, I scribbled key words for each question and then wrote rapidly, watching the time to divide it into five equal time blocks. I shortchanged the fifth question. Two hours later, I left the exam exhausted.

When the test was handed back, the professor said, "I'm going to read three of the best answers. Those that pulled from all the various sources."

Great, I thought. *Now, I'll learn what a good answer ought to be.*

The first two answers went on and on. I heard obscure tidbits I remembered, but only vaguely. For sure, here was evidence that my brain capacity was too limited for doctoral work. By the time the prof started reading the third answer, I had slid down in my armchair desk, deflated. Soon, however, his words began to sound familiar. I listened harder. The answer was *mine*. I worked hard not to grow red. I was almost embarrassed. I can still feel the glow that filled my face. I looked around, slowly, to make sure the other students weren't looking at me.

I hardly needed my feet to float out of class. Afterwards, I worried much less about my ability to hack the intellectual challenges of the program.

As in my master's program, I needed to choose a research interest. Before starting the doctorate, I'd thought about studying leisure again, but the concept of stigma had intrigued me for some time. The patients I met on the psychiatric units often talked about how they felt ostracized due to their mental illness. They never wanted anyone to know that they were patients on a psychiatric unit. They had been told to pull themselves up by the bootstraps, that a mental illness was simply mind over matter, or that their relationship wasn't right with God.

I felt the same stigma as my patients. And, because I felt it, I had chosen over the years not to reveal my own history of a psychiatric hospitalization. It was not worth the risk of being thought "crazy" simply because I'd felt restless as a full-time mom in the early seventies.

Betty Friedan had agreed.

But I did want to find out more about stigma, so I engaged in an extensive computer search in the library to find articles. Within a week, I found hundreds—many more than I would ever be able to assimilate in the time I'd allotted myself for this doctorate. I felt too old, five years from fifty, to drag the school process out. I could explore this more after I'd earned the degree.

I returned to my love of Sadie, the subject in my master's research who gave me the plastic red rose in the water-filled, egg-shaped vase. Sadie, upset about how she spent her free time. Sadie, feeling like a dummy "going round and round" as she circled her nursing home. In that research I had asked my older subjects *how* they preferred to spend their free or leisure time, but not *why*. This time I planned to explore *why*. I wanted to know if their stated preferences were also their desires. I wanted to get at the meaning, the kind of satisfaction they got, of participating in each activity.

I couldn't imagine, at age ninety, sitting in a nursing home and having to spend my day in activities that would make me feel like a dummy. I'd tell my kids that if they ever had to put me in a nursing home, never to set me up at a table with Popsicle sticks and Elmer's glue, and that I'd only go to a nursing home as the Director of Nursing—I'd run the home from my wheelchair, if necessary.

Through my study, I hoped to contribute to the literature that caregivers would read to help make the lives of older persons as meaningful as possible.

Late that fall, Jon called with an announcement. "Mom, Sheri and I would like to get married. Probably on spring break. Would that work in your schedule?"

Why now, for Pete's sake? The busiest time of my life! How would I ever fit this into my frantic schedule? And, why did this come up, anyway? He wasn't that serious when he'd left for school a few months before. "They're only juniors," I said to Marv. "They can't possibly know what they want."

I recalled Jon's first phone call home, from nursery school at age four when he was learning our phone number. What a surprise that had been! To answer the phone mid-afternoon while I was reading and Kathleen was napping and hear, "Mommy?" I'd nearly exploded with happiness at the sound of my little boy's soft and tentative voice.

Now that same voice had been deep and assured. I came to my senses, but continued to argue with Marv. "They are way too young to get married. They're only twenty!"

"And how old were you when we got married?" His tone insinuated memory loss on my part.

"Twenty." Subject closed.

Others jumped in to plan our part of the wedding; I was simply too busy. The wedding was held in Seattle, Sheri's hometown. Two of my sisters lived there. Kay held a formal rehearsal dinner in her sprawling family room; Rose shopped Nordstrom for my lavender silk dress, coordinating jewelry, and cream-colored heels, hose, and purse. All Marv and I had to do was show up. My sister Esther, in Grand Rapids, found us a seamstress near Calvin to make Kathleen's bridesmaid dress. Marv's sister-in-law helped arrange a Michigan reception in her church's fellowship hall.

While my part of the wedding was being planned for me, I was working with my classmates to complete weekly statistics assignments in a computer lab. After class, one of us met with the TA, or teacher's assistant, to clarify the expectations of the assignment for the others in our small group. Then each of us in that group worked one type of problem and shared the results so all of us would be able to complete many different types of problems each week on time. It was not unusual to spend forty hours with my calculator to write out each step, pages and pages, to answer one question. I couldn't have survived without my classmates. I don't know how to do the statistical tests anymore, but I still savor their names rolling over my tongue: ANOVA, Multiple Regression, Factor Analysis…

In spring quarter, I got one theories presentation out of the way before the wedding, choosing a topic I neither knew nor cared anything about simply because it was assigned to be presented first. For the second one, I signed up for Orem's self-care deficit theory. It certainly helped that Marianna and I had giggled over the "S-C-A is less than T-S-C-D equals S-C-D" formula in our bachelor's program and that I had taught Orem's theory, subsequently, to my own students at Trinity. I could prepare for this in my sleep, which is about what I did.

My year's academic leave, 1987-88, passed in a haze of commuting, studying, writing papers, and planning for the leisure research project. Without Marianna, my library copy card became my constant companion. I spent hours standing by the machine, copying articles I'd need for my research that I'd be finishing during Trinity's school breaks and summers after I returned to work.

The summer of 1988, Kathleen came home from Calvin and worked in a specialty produce shop. I ambled up to meet her after work and the day-old, jelly-filled donuts she'd have for us from the shop next door. Jon reluctantly sent his bride to her home in Seattle and left to take eleven weeks of basic training as an Army reservist at Fort Sill, Oklahoma. Marv stayed steady in the background, supporting each of us and paying lots of bills. I completed my final coursework before I returned to teaching that fall. Our family of five reunited at Fort Sill to see Jon graduate in August. We were shocked, then proud of his "lean and mean" stature. My fist bounced off his arm, his chest, his stomach. He, for sure, was no longer my little boy.

That fall, on the eve of our twenty-sixth anniversary, Jon, Sheri, and Kathleen were safely back at Calvin, my coursework was completed, and I had only my dissertation to finish. Life was good.

Sixteen

FIRST SHOTS

rthopedic clinicals—a high speed marathon giving me a caffeine rush that reminded me happily of my early med-surg days at Blodgett. A great part of my fall teaching assignment after my year's academic leave for doctoral course work.

Teaching this clinical on an orthopedic unit was fun, but work. On Monday mornings, the day before a two-day stint, I spent two hours on an ortho unit to select the patients for the students' assignments. I got ideas from the unit manager or primary nurses or by flipping through the Kardex. Then, from the Kardex at the nurses' station and from med sheets in a notebook on a med cart in each of three hallways, I recorded, on a detailed grid I'd drawn, the patients' diagnoses, treatments, diagnostic tests, and medications. I used the grid for my review before the clinical and to use as a checklist during the clinical.

Mid-afternoon, after classes, the students went to the hospital to read their patient's chart, introduce themselves, and then go home or to their dorm room to spend four or more hours completing a care plan from the data they had gathered. They knew they had to come to clinical "safe to practice," a challenging task for our junior students in their first experiences caring for patients.

At seven the next morning, my group of eight students and I, fortified with free coffee, huddled around a corner table in the softly lit hospital cafeteria for pre-conference. I was proud of my students—they looked and acted professional in their white pantsuits with a navy strip down either side of the bodice. Other students meeting near us were wearing cobbler-apron tops in assorted colors that reminded me of waitresses. During our pre-conference, each student presented her patient, using initials only, explaining the diagnosis, tests, treatments, and the nursing care needed that day.

Winding up pre-conference at 7:00, I said, "Come to get me the minute your patient requests a pain shot. We'll try to give it within fifteen minutes." We took the elevator to the fourth floor where I'd assigned students to patients on the three wings that met at an intersection. Standing at the intersection, I said, "I'll see those of you on the south hall to set your meds up at 8:30, west hall at 8:45, and east hall precisely at 9:00. Have your med sheets out of the notebook on top of the med cart. Put your unit dose packets, unopened, on top of the name of the right med on the sheet." I looked around for questions. I saw only wide eyes that looked as though they were trying to appear calm. "Now you're on your own. Find your patient's primary nurse for report. Remember, when your patients say they want a nurse, *you're* the nurse!"

I could count on a student's patient needing a pain shot before I had time to make my first rounds. Giving a shot made these beginning students feel like a "real" nurse. So I made sure everyone gave at least one shot in the ten days we spent on the unit. Since antibiotics were now given by IV piggyback solutions, the shots were primarily intramuscular for pain, and less frequently for insulin or anticoagulants. They'd practiced giving shots in our nursing lab, using an orange or a specially purchased "injection pillow"—both simulated the puncture feel of entering skin and the resistance feel of injecting the "medication," which was either sterile water or sterile saline. They didn't have to practice on each other, like I had done in nurses' training. My classmates and I inched down our waist-high cotton underwear, careful to expose only the smallest portion of the "upper outer quadrant" of our buttock.

This day was no different. Tall, blonde, and doing a two-step, Jennifer caught up with me in the intersection. Breathlessly, she said, "My patient wants her pain shot." And this is where the theater began.

"Great, Jennifer! You get to give a shot! Do you have the narcotic keys yet?"

"No, I couldn't find the nurse who's carrying them," Jennifer said, trying to sound as if she did this routine every hour.

"One RN is in 420. Check with her." Then I reiterated the procedure students had learned in nursing lab. "After you have the keys, check the doctor's order sheet in the patient's chart to make sure the narcotic order is still within the valid three-day window. Also, check the patient's med sheet on the med cart to see the last time it was given—make sure it's not too soon to give another—and check where it was given. Remember, we rotate sites. I'll be in the narcotic room waiting for you in about five minutes."

At 8:07, Jennifer strode into the narcotic room, off the nurses' station, clutching the keys as if they were diamonds. I was waiting, hands in the pockets of my lab coat that I wore over a pink mock turtleneck and gray slacks. Keeping my hands in my pockets reminded me not to grab the syringe myself because, of course, I could prepare the shot much faster.

"What do you need to do first?" I asked.

"Wash my hands. Find the right size syringe and needle."

"Which is what?"

"A 23 gauge, 1 ½ inch."

"Great. Good start. Now open the cupboard. It's always double-locked. Play with the keys to figure out which ones work."

The door swung open to display two shelves crowded with boxes of vials, ampules, and cartridges. I stood between Jennifer and the doorway, hoping to shut out any distraction from the hurry scurry of doctors and nurses in the nurses' station.

"What am I looking for?" Jennifer asked.

"That medicine comes in a vial."

Another four minutes passed as Jennifer found the right med; checked the number of vials left in the box with the number signed out on the corresponding narcotic sheet; replaced the box; locked both doors; and signed the sheet with the patient's name, room number, doctor's name, drug, dose, and her name. As an RN, I needed to co-sign her signature for narcotics.

It was 8:11.

Jennifer picked up the syringe and stopped short. "I can't do it. I'm shaking too much."

"Yes, you can. Take a deep breath. Shake your arms loose. Here, let's do flopsies together." I stood back from the counter and did a dance with my shoulders and arms and hands. She gingerly laid the syringe on the counter, giggled, and complied.

I turned and peeked out the door to make sure no one was watching. In the hallway, across the half-wall of the station, a nursing administrator was walking by. She briefly glanced our way. I hoped my department chair would not be getting a call about an instructor behaving unprofessionally on the unit.

When Jennifer was all flopsied loose, she carefully followed procedure and withdrew the exact amount of medication. After she flicked out teeny air bubbles, she held the syringe at eye level for me to check. "It's exactly at the 1cc mark, isn't it? Flush with the black line?"

"Yes, it is. I told you that you could do it!" I said, checking my watch. 8:14. "What will you say when we get to the room?"

As we walked side by side down the hallway, Jennifer, carrying the syringe on a small aqua plastic tray as though the filled syringe were a best actress award, answered, "I'm ready to give you your shot."

"How will you say it?" I prompted.

"Confidently!" Jennifer smiled.

"What will you do next?"

Jennifer's eyes rolled upward, as if picturing the page in her skills book. Sentences popped out of her mouth. "I'll check her name band. Then I'll help her roll to her left side since the last shot was given on her right. Then I'll locate the bony landmarks on her buttock to determine the appropriate injection site. Then I'll swab the area in circular motion with an alcohol pad. Then I'll take the cap off my syringe...without pricking myself. And then Ill tell her she will feel a prick."

"Wow, you're sounding like your skills book!" I laughed. "You've really got this memorized. Good for you."

At the bedside, syringe in hand, Jennifer said, "You will now feel a prick," then hesitated mid-air. Standing on the other side of the bed, I nodded and said with my eyes, "You can do this." As her syringe barely scratched the skin surface—something about puncturing the skin for the first time gave students the heebie-jeebies—I took my right hand off the patient's hip and gently pushed Jennifer's wrist down so the needle would go down to its hub.

Back in the hallway at 8:20 (great timing for a first shot), Jennifer's eyes twinkled. "I did it! I didn't even faint!" She sounded like she'd landed the star role in a Broadway play. And I had finished with her in time to start the rounds of the 8:30, 8:45, and 9:00 med cart rendezvous with the students.

The thrill of witnessing a student's "firsts" was the payoff that balanced the humor and energy and vigilance demanded of a clinical instructor. With eight beginning students, each caring for one patient, I was responsible for the safety of sixteen people, fewer than the twelve students and twelve patients I'd had in my first teaching job at Prairie State, but then some of the patients were in the hospital only for tests. Now patients who were admitted were always "sick" and needing complicated care.

My goal was to have a fun day for the students, but when "safety to practice" issues were at stake, it wasn't always possible. Each student had to arrive on time. She had to come with her newfound knowledge documented on a care plan. And she had to be able to answer questions underlying her patient care. No matter how gentle I tried to be in dealing with these issues when they occurred, I know the student had no fun. And I didn't either. Those were the nights when I would listen to the Rose of Sharon branches scratch our bedroom window in the wind and try to figure out what I could've done differently. I didn't want to be the one to crush any student's dream of becoming a nurse.

The morning passed quickly. My routine included making multiple unobtrusive rounds to observe each student; they knew I might be right outside a curtain or door. And supervising them in such skills as assessing their patients, giving baths, making beds (often "occupied beds" with patients in them draped in bulky dressings and immobilizing devices), changing dressings, inserting catheters, applying TED hose, monitoring IVs, and, of course, passing meds. Add supervising the few insulin and anticoagulant shots to the pain shots, and the five-hour morning made my body feel like I'd run the Boston marathon on hospital tiles.

In all my years of teaching clinicals, my students never made a med error. I was happy about this. But then it could not have happened because I was meticulous about watching them follow the "five rights" of medication administration: right med, right dose, right route of administration, right time, and right patient.

During post-conference at 11:30 in a small room on the unit, each student gave report on her morning. Jennifer blurted: "I gave my first shot. I guess you all know that by now!" The rest laughed. Everyone rejoiced in each other's accomplishments. And, carefully tracing her finger down her written care plan, Jennifer reported, "I took care of A.J., a seventy-two-year-old white female who had a left hip replacement yesterday for degenerative joint disease. She's a patient of Dr. Markin. Vitals were stable; bowel sounds weak, but present; she's sipping clear liquids and her IV is running at a keep open rate. Foley catheter was patent and draining clear yellow; left hip dressing was dry and intact so it didn't need reinforcement; Hemoglobin and Hematocrit were normal—she had one unit of blood during surgery. I reapplied her SCDs [Sequential Compression Devices] on her legs after her bath before log rolling her on her side. Some of you guys know this, because you and Dr. Roelofs were there to help me. My patient said we really cheered her up today. Oh, and she did her incentive spirometry treatments—ten times—every hour, so she shouldn't get any lung complications."

In a language that was foreign only weeks before, students now spoke with assurance. I could not help but feel proud of them, the same fireworks pride I'd had myself as a student when I'd learned to say, without stumbling, the surgical procedure "choledochojejunostomy."

Over lunch with a colleague, after getting our fatigue complaints out of the way, we'd always agree that the most fun of clinical teaching was to be there when the student did a new skill for the first time. To feel their excitement. To see the spark in their eyes. To be able to say, "You did a great job!"

And now I would like to let my former ortho students know that I missed them terribly in 2006 when I became an orthopedic patient with a fractured hip from a fall. I know they would not have "fished" around pre-op to insert my Foley catheter that most certainly contributed to a post-op urinary tract infection. I could have used their help to log roll myself from side to side to grab my ringing phone that was left out of my reach. I would have enjoyed their humor as I lay immobilized by the compression devices on my legs, the catheter burning in place, and an IV stinging in my arm. And I would have liked to hear their jokes on how this mishap could have happened to me, the person that used to be the teacher, the woman standing at the side of the bed, not lying in it.

Seventeen

NOTHING PHYSICAL

ear casual street clothes that can be washed, with flat shoes or clean tennis shoes. Do not wear jeans (any color), spandex, stirrup pants, dangly earrings, or anything that can be interpreted as unprofessional."

Students loved getting out of their uniforms and wearing street clothes for the mental health nursing clinical that I taught every spring while at Trinity. I had to add the "any color" to the "do not wear jeans" direction in the syllabus because a student came once on the first day in regular blue jeans. When I reminded her, she came the next day in green jeans, and then the third day in red jeans. Nice enough jeans, but the telltale seaming and rear pockets screamed "jeans" to our clinical agency.

My major concern was students' fear of the unknown. They had preconceived notions of what a psychiatric unit would be like (people hanging from chandeliers was a common one), most of which would be dispelled by the end of the first clinical day, especially if staff had mistaken them for patients. With students wearing street clothes, staff sometimes didn't see their first-name-only badges and would ask them who their assigned nurse was, or tell them they needed to attend their group meeting, or warn them to get out of another patient's room.

Students were then impressed with their own similarities to some of the patients.

A typical clinical day started at 8:00 a.m., listening to the PM and night taped reports with just our student group. *Jonas Berzinsky is in for depression. He's on EPs and SPs.* Using the pause button, I asked questions: "What are EPs?" Elopement precautions. "What are SPs?" Suicide precautions. *The doctor may start him on Lithium today.* Pause button. "What is Lithium usually given for?" Bipolar disorder. "Why would this patient be going on Lithium?" Maybe depression was the admitting diagnosis, but we'll find symptoms of mania or hypomania documented on the chart. "What is the normal therapeutic range of Lithium?" Around 1 mEq per liter. Point 6 to 1.4. (They'd put up their index finger like I had showed them in class to remember the "one" when taking state boards. This blood level was sure to be a question.) "What are side effects?" Fine hand tremor, polyuria, polydipsia.

If there was no patient with schizophrenia on the unit on a particular day, I asked, "What behaviors would you expect to see in schizophrenia?" I gave an acronym I'd learned or made up years earlier: P-TAM. Changes in perception, thought, affect, and mood.

From the taped report, students selected a patient with whom they wanted to do a "one-to-one." I allowed them to pick their own patients to make sure they stayed comfortable. I soon found they often picked the patient that intimidated them the most. After we left the report room, they introduced themselves to their patients, explained their student status, and asked to talk with them some time that day. They followed a process they had learned of helping patients identify their concerns and explore solutions.

My goal for the students was for them to become more aware of how they related to patients. I wanted them to feel the notion of "therapeutic use of self"—to know they were their own best tool when talking with a patient. And, along the way, to become comfortable with people who were experiencing alcohol and drug abuse, depression and bipolar disorder, and schizophrenia.

Giving meds was not a concern on a psychiatric unit. None of our agencies allowed us to give meds because students wouldn't have had the experience to assess subtle side effects or to observe if patients were "cheeking" their pills when they didn't want to take them.

Depending on what groups were available—activity therapy, group therapy, education seminars, or art therapy—each student attended at least one group per day. If possible in the setting, students shadowed the chaplain for a day. A usual response was, "I can't believe how quickly every single patient opened up to the chaplain. The chaplain somehow has instant rapport." As they heard patients talk with the chaplain, they noted how closely spiritual issues dovetailed with emotional concerns: "If God truly loves me, why is it I'm depressed? Why doesn't He make it go away? What have I done to cause this?" And they noted how easily the chaplain was able to reassure the patients that God didn't cause the disease, even though it might feel like it at times.

During free time, students read charts and mingled in dayrooms, playing board games or coloring with the patients. When students were in groups or involved with their patients, I, too, colored many pages from coloring books over the years, all the while carrying on informal conversations with patients. "What brought you to the hospital?"

An older woman, tangled bleached hair falling over her eyes, said, "Couldn't handle it anymore. My husband died last year. We'd been married fifty-four years. Kids don't care about me." She pressed down harder on her crayon. Her chipped nails had been painted dark red. "They never come by. The house is so still. And I've got this arthritis. It all got to be too much."

"Uh huh. Sounds like a lot to handle by yourself…how's it going for you here?" I continued to concentrate on my coloring. Patients talked readily when I didn't look at them.

"Oh, it's slow, but I am feeling better. Joe, that leader in group, is so good, He makes us state goals each day, even tiny ones, like put lipstick on. And I do it, and I feel better. And it makes me feel better to talk to those students of yours, too. They are such nice girls. And there's one young man, too, isn't there? They seem so interested in me. And I loved the pets yesterday. That one kitty came right to me. It reminded me of when I lived on the farm as a little girl. So soft, warm, purring away…"

I saw my role during the psychiatric clinical as fostering the physical and emotional safety of each student. Teaching them safety measures: don't sit with your back to patients; sit by the door in a small locked unit; never try to restrain a patient—call for help. Being alert when student emotions began to shake and taking the student off the unit to defuse in a safe place. Sometimes a student discovered that an acquaintance was a patient and would not know how to deal with it. More likely, a patient reminded a student of an unhappy experience—like an alcoholic parent—and the student would need to talk about the pain. I recall one student saying, "I thought I'd worked it all through. I haven't seen my dad in years. I thought it was over. But the patient's smell, his boots, and his loud slurred speech made growing up with alcohol all come back. Will this ever end?"

There were a few students over the years who reached the point of suicidal thoughts or attempts. Too many painful issues surfaced too quickly. My mentor Maureen back at Prairie State had warned me when it first happened there. I was glad because it was natural as a psych nurse to want to listen, to help, but as years passed I became better at identifying students who seemed likely to have problems and referring them to the college counseling services. I also became better at conveying to the students that my role was teacher, not counselor. That their role was student, not patient. That the course was education, not therapy.

Locked doors added to the intensity of the emotional content of each day. Students needed to ask me for the key to the bathroom or to leave the unit. I tried to lighten the mood a little by reminding them I was their only clinical instructor who also got to know their bathroom habits (and their early morning on-the-way-to-clinical coffee habits), and they'd better be nice to me or they might not get to lunch in the cafeteria.

They soon learned to go to the bathroom in tandem.

At the end of each clinical day, we had an hour's post-conference. The students presented the patient with whom they'd had their one-to-one, carefully protecting confidential information. One said, "My patient told me all about how her husband beat her. I had told her right away that I wouldn't be sharing any details with you guys of what she said, but I would have to give a report to her primary nurse." They described their experiences attending groups, applying group dynamic theory to roles they saw staff and patients play, such as being an encourager or monopolizer. Exactly what I'd learned in my master's program. They also shared their informal conversations with patients in the dayroom, applying what they'd learned from their textbook and lectures. "One woman told me she felt like she was spitting cotton. I checked her meds and two were dryer-uppers—I mean they had anticholinergic side effects—like the chart in the book showed, so I was able to explain to her this may be causing her dry mouth."

I loved teaching theory-based nursing, and in these post-conferences the students' reports played inspiring background music in my mind.

Sometimes students had to laugh. One student tried her best not to have her voice break: "My patient thought she was a bird. It was so hard to do my one-to-one with her, because she kept bobbing her head down on the table, like a woodpecker." The other students looked at me to see if it was okay to let go of their shock with a giggle. I explained, "That's why we have ample time in post-conference in psych. We see behaviors and hear stories that are new to us—which understandably are amusing—especially at first. We can laugh here where we can desensitize ourselves."

More often, though, students would feel the patients' emotional pain. The difficult family situations and deep personal hurts that patients had shared with them during the day frequently cast the post-conference group into a gray mood that matched the Midwestern winter days of this clinical. Students said they often napped when they got home "even though we did nothing physical all day like we do in the other clinicals." Many reported that they would be calling their folks to tell them "thanks" for bringing them up in a loving, supportive home. They learned to appreciate the pain of mental illness. They learned not only to care for the patients, but to care about them as individuals.

As I listened to their intense emotions, I'd think that even if none of them ever worked in a psychiatric setting, if each one would help meet the emotional needs of only one person a week, thousands would be helped over a lifetime.

Eighteen

FANCY TITLE

I didn't look for another job; a nurse recruiter called me, a person I'd worked with to find jobs for students, to tell me of openings for new grads. In our conversation, I told her I'd recently finished my dissertation and graduated. She said, "Oh, now that you're done with your PhD, I have a position I think you may be interested in."

A research position at a major medical center. With doctors. Why not look into it? It was 1991, and I was already forty-nine. If I was going to sew wild oats yet, maybe this was the time.

I made up my mind a few weeks later during a clinical when all my students were involved in groups, and I was sitting alone in a dayroom. I'd been back at Trinity for three years since my academic leave and my head said it was time to try something new. Settling into an empty consult office, I called my academic dean at the college. "I've decided to take another job…." There was no way of knowing then that I'd work in three places holding four positions during the next five years. Would that have made a difference in my decision? No.

Four months later, I burst into tears as Marv moved boxes out of my faculty office. Eight years of memories—months of teaching experiences, weeks of curriculum work, immeasurable amounts of physical and emotional time. *So much of me was there.*

My body, as filled with emotion as my boxes were with books, felt as if it would burst.

It took only a few weeks to know I'd made the wrong decision. I had a fancy title for an unfancy job—assisting a psychiatrist with his research, the doctor with whom I'd interviewed and on a topic that interested me at the time.

Dr. Patel was cordial and respectful, and our joint office was roomy, though old. Two double-hung windows, thirty-two panes apiece, looked out on other red brick medical buildings and the short roadway to the VA hospital where Marianna worked in home care. Being near Marianna helped me decide to take this job.

And, at first, I liked scheduling my own time, twenty hours a week, and diddling long hours in the library doing literature searches for Dr. Patel. After doing my own dissertation, I was relieved to do the almost mindless work.

But by early fall, I found myself sitting close to visitors in the cafeteria to have conversations. "What brings you to the hospital?" I'd ask over pizza, savoring every stressful detail of their story. When I started plotting how I could trip visitors on my way to the library so I could touch them, I realized, once again, that by taking a paper-oriented job, I was missing people. I wondered if I'd ever learn.

I not only missed the fun of my students, but, working in my male-dominated, physician-only department, I missed nurses. I was thrilled when the chief psychiatrist arranged for me to work one day a week assisting Sherry, the bachelor's prepared research nurse assigned to assist the doctors with their projects.

We both worked on a study of serial killers. It was fun meeting her to go to the monthly meetings of the research team where we listened to reports from an FBI profiler and forensic psychiatrists. After many lone hours in the library, I felt like a voyeur picturing shootings and stranglings and executions. And, after years of serving on nursing curriculum committees, I found the topic of serial killers to be much more exciting than the latest testing strategies.

At lunch I no longer had to accost visitors. I had Sherry to go to lunch with, and she and I talked about our respective literature searches. She'd say, "Did you know vampires used to hang people upside down in cages spiked with nails and watch them bleed to death?"

I'd say, "No way," my eyes bulging as I imagined the bodies of moaning, emaciated men dripping blood in big blobs on an asphalt tile floor. "All I've been reading about is body parts being stored in refrigerators and buried under basement floors." As I talked, I saw Mason jars in my mind, lined up on the top shelf of a fridge, filled with pickled pigs' feet.

I ate happily through our body-dismantling discussions.

In the afternoon of the days I worked with Sherry, I helped her interview patients at the VA for a gambling study. The subjects' faces lit up as they described the first rush they got from gambling. For many, it was while playing craps in the alleyways behind their houses. I felt warm and relaxed being back with patients and hearing their stories. When our interviews were finished for the day, Sherry served me tea in her office at the VA and we gabbed. Those times, and seeing Marianna, were some of the best times I had on that job.

Once every two weeks or so, I'd go next door to Marianna's office to wait for her while she finished up calls for her next day's appointments. We'd go for dinner and compare notes. She'd tell me of her home visits: "I saw five people today, all dying." I pictured her in those homes dealing with patients in pain and families in mourning. I became envious. She, with a master's degree, seemed to have a far more fulfilling job than I did with my doctorate.

What was wrong with me? I'd been happy to give up responsibility for my own research, students, and faculty work, but now was feeling a huge emptiness. How had I gotten myself here? I clearly hadn't comprehended what my job would be. And I was unable to articulate to the doctors what my capabilities as a nurse with a doctorate were.

I didn't even know myself. I didn't even respond when Dr. Patel amiably suggested I add a piece of my own interests to projects I was working on with him. I fell into playing the subservient role I'd learned so well. I hoped I wasn't forever rooted in my diploma school mentality after all.

Late fall, I overheard a psychiatrist outside my office talking about needing co-therapists for couples using the medical center's sexual dysfunction treatment services. Eager to see more patients, I jumped out of my office chair to inquire.

After a day-long orientation, I volunteered as a co-therapist from 5:00 to 10:00 one night a week for seven weeks, followed by another seven-week session. All day I looked forward to 4:00, when I could mosey over to the clinic. I wondered what sexual dysfunction I would be working with, female or male. It turned out that the couple in each of my sessions was dealing with male impotence. I heard about elaborate plans for affairs, vacuum pumps for erectile difficulties, and the day-to-day frustrations of neither partner knowing how to cure the problem. Sitting in a small consultation room hearing the intimate stories, I loved feeling like a real nurse again and was pleased I could help.

I was not pleased, however, with my co-therapist, a cardiac surgeon. An older man, he was volunteering at the clinic to earn his required continuing education units. The coordinator who matched up co-therapists said that I, as a nurse, would be able to handle him. I didn't know what that meant, but I soon found out. After being a delightful person to work with for the first four hours, he would get a phone call at the beginning of the fifth and final hour. There were no cell phones then, so a staff person would come to the door and tell him he had an urgent call. He'd quickly appear flustered and tell me he had to leave; something important needed his attention.

I wondered how many urgent calls could happen at precisely the same time on the same evening every week. I soon suspected he only wanted to get home on time. I felt again like a doctor go-fer. I had to meet with the couple during the final hour on my own, which, in spite of feeling stranded, I thoroughly enjoyed. I actually felt the couple was more open with me alone than when the surgeon was there.

One morning in the spring, Dr. Patel told me of the possibility that we would be relocated to another psychiatric facility to conduct a major research project, something to do with schizophrenia. My future dropped like a black stage curtain in front of my eyes. I asked if the job would be full-time—I was ready for full-time again—and about salary. He said his would be about $125,000; mine, if my hours could be increased to full-time, would be about $40,000. That was less than I'd made for a nine-month year teaching. I blew, diplomatically, of course: "That is not fair."

He, always the gentleman, smiled. "I know, Lois. But life is not fair. Think of what a plumber gets paid. And he doesn't even have a PhD."

I started looking for another job.

Late spring, Marianna told me of an opening at her VA hospital for a psychiatric nurse educator. I ran over to pick up the application. To teach, to work with nurses, to work in the same place as Marianna again—I was ecstatic. I waltzed through the complex interview process, passed the mandatory pharmacology test, and eagerly awaited the day I could call for my start date. On that day, I called the chief nurse. As the phone rang, I looked out my window and saw the short roadway to the new building where I would be working. I would have my own office, soft blue with modern modular furniture. No old beat up desk. The chief nurse answered, "I don't know how to tell you. I just got out of a meeting in which my educator position was cut. I'm terribly sorry."

I called Marianna. Tearing up my resignation letter, I plunged into a blue funk that lasted into the summer.

The job section of the Sunday *Chicago Tribune* became my Bible. In July, at last, I saw an ad for a psychiatric nursing faculty member, PhD preferred, at Valparaiso University in Indiana. I immediately called a friend whose son went there. "How long a drive is it?"

"About an hour, easy driving," she assured me.

I interviewed on July 15, 1992. The dean offered me the position. I sailed home up Ripley Street to 94 to 294 to find a message on our answering machine. "Congratulations, Grandma!" In Seattle, Jon and Sheri had had their first child, Kristin Kathleen. Kathleen, after our daughter. I thought of all the times Jon and Kath had fought as little kids—she was always mad that she would always be two years younger and would have to wait for the newest privilege. He would tease her—and now he had named his firstborn after her.

Too many good things had happened to me that day. Waiting for Marv, the new Grandpa in our family, to come home from work, I got out of my interview suit, threw on jeans, slumped into my favorite blue recliner, and let the tears flow down my face.

Nineteen

NO SURPRISES, BE LEGAL

*B*arely a month later, I sat in my new office at Valparaiso University and watched laughing college students walk by. My enthusiasm matched theirs. The camaraderie among the female faculty, diverse student body, and two-person office staff in the College of Nursing erased any concerns I had over the one-hour commute from Palos Heights.

My teaching load consisted of an orientation-type semester—at full pay: just two clinical sections of eleven students each, plus auditing a psychiatric nursing theory course so I could teach it the next semester. Because morning clinicals started early, I treated myself to dinner, a barbeque sandwich and root beer float at Al's Diner, and stayed overnight at a Super 8, enjoying my interruption-free evening propped up in bed grading care plans.

A few weeks into the semester, a colleague became ill, and I was assigned to teach the theory course and take on a third clinical group. Teaching three groups involved going to two psychiatric facilities. I graded thirty-three care plans weekly and the same number of thirty-page case studies at the end of the semester.

Clinicals were only four hours long. We started and finished each clinical with a half-hour conference. Between conferences, students attended one or two groups and talked one-to-one with at least one patient. As required by the syllabus, I methodically conducted half-hour oral med quizzes with each student during the clinical. Doing two on each clinical day enabled me to finish each group of eleven in five to six weeks. The four hours raced by.

I thrived on the new pace of my life.

The theory class consisted of sixty-seven students, all with a previous bachelor's degree in other fields and life experience, unlike my younger students at Trinity. One gal in her thirties told me, "I'm being stalked by an old boyfriend. Don't worry if he shows up. The police are on it." Another said, "Don't tell anyone. I'm embarrassed. But I'm out of money and living in my car." A police officer told the class of abuse cases: "You think it's only women who get abused. Not true! I answered a husband's call once and this woman comes flying out and nails me in the gut with the spike heel she's clutching in her hand." A speech therapist convinced us nursing was more fulfilling: "A nurse gets to do more than I do; she works with every age group, works with every part of the body, works in every type of setting in the hospital and the community, and can work every hour of the day, seven days a week." A mother of six wanted to graduate college with her oldest child: "I'm gonna show 'em that I'm as smart as they are!" She did. She went on to become a nurse practitioner.

One day with this enjoyably interactive class, I excitedly made an announcement that, after great difficulty finding a date, I had been able to schedule a fieldtrip to the state psychiatric hospital. Expecting all of them to be jubilant also, I was flabbergasted after class when three or four women angrily approached me. "We can't go. We have to register that day or we won't get the classes we need to graduate."

Rather than clarify their problem, I cavalierly said, "Oh, that's no problem. We'll be back before registration closes."

They responded, voices jumping off the walls, "We have to get there *first*, or the courses we need to take will be closed, and we won't be able to graduate."

I had never experienced seniors not being able to get required courses. And I should not have assumed I knew how registration worked there. We worked it out, but the situation certainly humbled me. I learned to ask more questions and not answer glibly without being sure I knew what I was talking about. One of the more vocal students surprised me on the next clinical day. Sitting on a couch awaiting the students, I was still shaken and not eager to face her again. When she burst in, she broke into a big grin and said, "It's always such a comfort to see you here waiting for us. This clinical makes me so nervous and just looking at you calms me down."

I could've hugged her. The uncertainty, I decided, is part of the fun of teaching. Never knowing what to expect (including my being asked to more than double my teaching load on a moment's notice) and never having to worry about being bored.

My dean, however, wanted to know what to expect. I admired her straightforward approach. She'd say, "I don't want my phone ringing to tell me you're doing something you shouldn't be doing, or to tell me you're saying something you shouldn't be saying. I want to know everything upfront." Her motto "no surprises, be legal" covered any questions I had about my work with the students, both in clinical and in the classroom. I took no chances; any complaint from an agency about us, any complaint from a student, I passed it on to her.

Midyear, she sent me to a conference in San Antonio on graduate education. "That's where I see you next year, Lois. Teaching in our graduate program." She'd already assigned me to teach an independent study in family therapy for one graduate student that was giving me a chance to teach material I'd had in my own master's coursework. It was good to recall my own family visits, including the family with the cats, dogs, cockroaches, incest, and no goals, and to remember how my colleague and I had been able to make an impact that showed we cared. I looked forward to going to the conference. My sister Kay, now a dean of a graduate nursing program in the Midwest, would be going too. We could catch up strolling along the River Walk and rolling our tongues over hot fudge sundaes.

At the conference, I met the nursing dean from St. Xavier, a university near my home. "What are you doing now, Lois?... Really, driving that far? Keep your eyes open; I may have an administrative opening soon. Watch the newspapers."

I anxiously reported this possibility to my dean. The university had paid for my conference, I was looking forward to teaching in the graduate program, and now I might have an opportunity to leave. I had no need to worry. She'd said earlier, with my PhD, I should be teaching in a graduate program or going into administration. Now she said, matter-of-factly, "If you think you'd like to try administration, go for it and get it out of your system."

So what did I want to do? Continue commuting an hour and teach in the graduate program? Or maybe cut that commute down to fifteen minutes and try administration? Just like after earning my bachelor's, and then my master's, with the PhD, I now had more options to consider.

Driving west on my commutes home, I watched the brilliance of a slowly developing orange sunset while listening to triumphal hymns on WMBI, the Moody Bible Institute station. My spirits would soar when I'd happen to hear "Majesty." One line reminded me of one of my dissertation subjects who'd said he did "everything to the honor and glory of God." The hour's drive gave me lots of time to pray about whether I should change jobs after only one year.

Twenty

SISTER MARY HOLY WATER

Coming from a Protestant background, do you think you'll be comfortable with us?"

I'm sure I had a startled look when I heard these words from the nursing dean, Pat Hemp, at St. Xavier University. I couldn't imagine asking that kind of question at Trinity, where some of my former nursing colleagues, minorities among the mostly Dutch, Christian Reformed faculty, would be shocked. I thought of when I listened to them bristle after someone in a college faculty meeting would espouse the Reformed worldview, unintentionally implying something derogatory about other beliefs. I would hurt for them and try to soothe.

So, naturally, I was greatly impressed, actually shocked, that Pat Hemp was concerned about my comfort as the outsider.

It had been a bit bumpy getting to this meeting. After talking with Pat in San Antonio in December of 1992, I scanned our regional *Nursing Spectrum* for weeks waiting to see what position she'd be advertising. When I finally saw the ad for an assistant dean for undergraduate nursing, a twelve-month position, I was excited to explore it.

I applied and was invited for an interview with faculty. We met in the nursing lab in the School of Nursing. I hadn't expected serious-looking faces and couldn't figure out how a room full of women could be so quiet. After whatever speech I gave, they asked few questions. I could've been at a wake. Maybe I was too cocky, too self-assured, because I didn't need this position.

Driving home, I had an uneasy feeling. I recalled Marianna's advice. She interviewed for jobs much more often than I did and had a mantra: "Trust your gut." I discussed the interview with Marv. He didn't know what to make of my recent jaunts from job to job, so he grinned and responded with his usual words, "I know you'll do what you want to anyway, so it doesn't really matter what I say."

A few days later I called and withdrew my application. If I stayed at VU, I could stay on a nine-month contract and teach in the graduate program. Then Pat Hemp called. "I heard you're no longer interested in our position. Can we meet for lunch to talk?"

Now we were sitting at a Hilton restaurant with a green and white trellis décor. A short woman, my age, with dark curly hair, Pat shared a long friendly lunch with me. I don't remember telling her that I'd withdrawn my application because I'd sensed something wrong from the mood of the room. But when she showed interest in my comfort in their Catholic culture, my misgivings began melting away. "I'm sure there'd be no problem," I said. "I've worked at a Catholic hospital, both as a clinical instructor when I was at Prairie State, and then as their nursing education coordinator. Except for the time I politely told a head nurse she had a smudge on her forehead on the first Ash Wednesday I worked there, I was comfortable."

We both laughed. I accepted the position.

My picture made the August 12, 1993, Palos Heights *Regional News.* I'm sitting at my new desk dressed in a mulberry linen blazer over a matching print dress. My short ash-blonde hair features a newly-permed, loose curly look. Behind my tortoise-rimmed glasses, I'm smiling.

I was thrilled to have the opportunity to be an assistant dean. After filling the acting chair position at Trinity nine years earlier, I had felt I did not need or want to be a dean. I did not want the ultimate responsibility. But I felt I could be a good sidekick. And I figured I could teach grad students later if I wished. And, right then, I was also happy to reduce my commute from fifty to eleven miles.

I looked forward to my new office; I loved making my little niches comfortable. I was given the largest office I'd ever had—about twelve feet square. It had room for a desk, credenza, conference table, several chairs, and file cabinets. There was even a free corner, so I bought a six-foot-tall ficus plant. The two windows flanked my desk and faced south—103rd St. The room was blue and soft and cozy, especially in the afternoon sun. The walls provided a pretty contrast to my burgundy-matted master's and PhD diplomas I had framed myself under guidance at a do-it-yourself shop.

As I read manuals and folders and memos related to my new responsibilities—approximately twenty undergraduate faculty and 500 students—I was pleasantly surprised by the faculty who stopped in to greet me. A few good-naturedly christened me the resident Dutch Protestant. "I think she must have a windmill in her front yard," one told another. "Most Dutch people do."

Faculty also ribbed me for the cotton throw I'd bought to drape over the armchair next to my desk. I'd seen it displayed at Penney's and couldn't resist the pattern—a bed of large teal and peach tulips on a white background. I hadn't thought of the Dutch connection being significant when I bought it.

There was a lighthearted sense of camaraderie in and out of my office, and I no longer felt the qualms I'd had after my interview. I hoped I would catch on quickly to the work and be able to make a difference. I knew they were ready for stability because there had been three people in the position in the four years before me.

I was determined to fit into the Irish Catholic setting—tulips, windmills, blonde hair, and all. A few weeks after I started, I got my first challenge. The dean told me to meet her the next morning at Queen of Martyrs. I had no idea what this meant, and she was gone before I could ask. I gave myself a Twenty Questions quiz. Person, place, or thing? Face cards came to mind: Queen of Hearts…Spades…Clubs…Diamonds. No Queen of Martyrs.

I didn't want anyone to know I didn't know. So when Vivian, my secretary, asked if I needed help with anything, I said, "Yes. Tomorrow morning. Queen of Martyrs. Where do I park?"

"Right in back of this building. Where you park now. You can walk across."

Great, that was helpful. Queen of Martyrs was a place, across something. But what? A bridge? The parking lot? The street?

When I left work that day, I spotted the Queen of Martyrs sign at a church across the street. I sighed with relief. I could save face, but not for long.

At Queen of Martyrs, I sat in a pew among other nursing faculty and watched a priest doing something on a table in front of the altar. A soloist sang responses to the priest's words. Her soprano was clear, full, flute-like. *Christ has died, Christ is risen, Christ will come again.* The sound of her voice made me think of heaven. My own churches had always had choirs, so the loveliness of this lone ethereal voice landed right in my heart and left me mesmerized.

A slam, crunch, ouch shook me out of my reverie. My colleagues fell to their knees. I couldn't move. I didn't know what was happening and felt my pulse act up. Leaning forward to check my toes, I saw the fronts of my black flats snuggly wedged beneath the kneeler. I'd forgotten about kneelers from the one time I'd been in a Catholic church to attend a wedding years before. Embarrassed, I wiggled my feet loose, one-eighth inch at a time.

A few others were also sitting, not kneeling. I tried to act as if nothing had happened.

By late fall when snow laced the branches outside my windows, I felt settled into my office and comfortably adapted to the Irish Catholic milieu. But I should've known not to get too smug. One afternoon after her clinical, Colette, a med-surg teacher, rushed through my doorway, "Hey, do you have a minute? I've got a problem."

Colette was an experienced teacher, my age. I was pleased she felt free to drop in and thought I could help her. "Sure, have a seat." I motioned her to sit down on my tulip field.

"I have a student who was a no show, no call, today in clinical. I couldn't reach her by phone. The same thing happened last week. I talked to her in class after that. She assured me it wouldn't happen again. What do you think?" She laughed, bright eyes twinkling. She leaned forward, "Do you think this is a situation for St. Jude?"

St. Jude. I had not encountered saints there, yet. Did I have to play Twenty Questions again? Has to be a person, I thought. I did not want to blow this woman's confidence in me, so drew on my psych background to ask an open-ended question: "I don't know. What do you think?"

"Well, I don't think she's a lost cause yet…"

I went to a Catholic bookstore and looked up St. Jude. A few weeks later, I confessed my ignorance to Colette and asked for a lecture on the saints. She invited me into her office and drew a map: Mother Teresa—step one—step two…

I got comfortable with stories of my colleagues' childhood experiences at new-to-me names of schools—St. Christina, St. Alexander, Mother McAuley—and with descriptions of nuns as teachers, wearing long swishing black habits and carrying rulers ready to tap little hands. Compared to Christian schools I'd attended, these sounded like they could be haunted mansions. "Watch out for the nuns. They're lurking everywhere, even in the cloakroom. They'll see if you are naughty or nice. They have rulers…."

My childhood schools were named unimaginatively after their location: West Sayville Christian, Lafayette Christian, Cutlerville Christian. Even adding a hint of gender in their names would add flavorful potential for storytelling. My teachers wore plaid straight skirts and plain nylon blouses. Nothing spooky. And they didn't have rulers. We got sent to sit in the hallway to repent of our sins. I sat there twice. The tile floor was cold—I pulled my knees to my chest and wrapped the skirt of my dress around my legs to keep warm.

Maybe a ruler-tap would have been warmer. Certainly quicker.

As it got close to St. Patrick's Day, I was excited to see exactly how it was celebrated. I'd heard lots about the South Side Irish and their ability to party. The day before, Barb, a younger faculty member, stopped in, "Wear green tomorrow. Gotta pretend you're Irish."

I wore green, but I hadn't anticipated the rest of learning to be Irish.

"Here, try this, Lois," Barb's friend, Paula, said at a faculty and staff celebration. "Irish coffee. It's sweet and got a zing."

We were seated at one of many round tables decorated with white tablecloths and shamrocks. I took the cup, smelled it, noted a strange odor, and drank a sip. "What's that taste?"

"A tad of Jameson. You won't even feel it."

I took a long large sip. The smooth liquid numbed my gums…warmed the journey to my stomach…sent lulling messages to my forehead.

"I see you've got her drinking the good stuff," Barb said as she arrived at the table with a plate heaped full of goodies. "Here, try a piece of Irish soda bread, too."

The bread looked like dried-out slices of pale-colored pound cake. I needed more Irish coffee to wash it down. The moistened cake was delicious. I dunked and ate a second piece.

Barb and Paula had to escort me back to my office—one on either side—down a long narrow tiled hallway. "You're not a good Irishman yet," Paula said. "Do you know the difference between an Irish funeral and an Irish wedding?"

I concentrated on my voice. *Make it sound level, strong,* I told myself, trying also not to giggle. "No, I don't."

"One less drunk."

I'd never heard that joke about Dutch folks. My parents never even had alcohol in the house. I was happy to be back safely ensconced in my swivel office chair with arms.

Soon after, Paula brought me a miniature bottle of Baileys Irish Cream. "Here, keep this in the back of a bottom desk drawer. Drink it at the end of a bad day."

I never did.

Shortly after St. Patrick's Day, I found a black collarless suit on sale. I wasn't thinking "nuns" when I wore it to work with a white mandarin-collared blouse, black hose, and black low-heeled pumps. When I opened the inside door to the nursing wing, I saw Colette, my sainthood teacher, scooting away from me toward her office. When the door whooshed shut behind me, she turned around, broke into an ear-to-ear smile, and shouted, "Sister Mary Holy Water."

"Who? What?" I said, laughing.

"In that black and white outfit, you look exactly like a nun. Sister Mary Holy Water! Now, for real, you fit right in around here."

I laughed. Her words affirmed my early determination to fit into the Irish Catholic setting. Her words were Irish Catholic music to my Dutch Protestant ears. Her words made me realize it was important for me to feel that I belonged.

Twenty-one

GETTING ORGANIZED

on't slide and fall," I would tell Vivian when she'd step over stacks of unsorted mail coming in for our 9:00 a.m. daily meetings. "I can't do without you!"

She'd laugh. "I'm used to it." A bit younger than I, Vivian wasn't easily fazed. It was my first time to have my own secretary and I often told her: "This job is a joint effort. With all your help, you make me look good."

And that was true. I would've had to paddle much harder to stay afloat without her.

I had plunged eagerly into my new work as an assistant dean. Each day reminded me of when I'd been acting chair at Trinity. In that job, the day's mail had taught me what I needed to do. Now, it wasn't only the mail, but the phone, and people at the door.

And meetings: deans meetings, faculty meetings, division directors meetings. And committees: standing committees, ad-hoc committees, university-wide committees. Each two hours long. I bumped into myself coming and going, gathering up agendas and folders between meetings. When I'd get back to my office for the day, I'd have a stack of items to add to my "to do" list.

I loved organizing—making sense of the dozens of tidbits that piled up in my six-by-nine-inch notebook. Between my excursions outside my office, I methodically addressed each item and checked it off as I completed it. I loved seeing piles of paper diminish. Often my office resembled the aftermath of a paper avalanche.

Early on, Vivian handed me a letter to sign saying to our agencies that all students were compliant with health requirements. In my previous three teaching positions, a secretary tracked these, so I asked Vivian for the tracking sheet. "There is none…yet," she said.

"What do you mean, yet?" She said a computerized tracking system had been talked about for awhile, but so far the office didn't have it, and they had not had time yet to do the hand tracking. To say I was surprised wouldn't cut it: I was flabbergasted. Students were due to start clinicals in a matter of days. I asked Vivian where the copies of the health requirements were. She told me that when the students brought them in, the office staff threw them in a big box under the counter. They were still in the box.

So, what was I to do? Assume everything was there and sign the letter? But could I assume that? What if a student transmitted a dread disease to a patient, and I couldn't provide proof that she'd had her shots?

I looked in the box and mentally calculated the number of pieces of paper—about 300 students in clinical, each having brought in a copy of their physical exam, immunizations, hepatitis series, rubella titer, TB test, and CPR certification. In the best picture, there might only be 300 pieces of paper; in the worst, I couldn't think about it. Just when gnawing pains as if I had fasted a month began attacking my stomach, a faculty member volunteered to organize the box full of slips of paper and set up a workable tracking system.

I hugged her in my mind. I would rest more easily when I knew things were taken care of properly, and I could act legally as my dean at VU had taught me. Now, I understood better her motto of "no surprises, be legal."

The tracking system of students' health requirements was only the beginning. I then tackled the three schedules around which my work revolved: faculty teaching assignments, courses offered, and clinical agency requests. None was on spreadsheet. Two were typed; one was handwritten landscape style on several sheets of oversized paper, color-coded with magic markers, reminding me of a fun kindergarten art project. When I spread out the various sheets of the three schedules on my rectangular conference desk, my linear mind saw a mile of messy jagged-edged columns of words. My head went helter-skelter trying to find order. How would I ever grasp the details of the job when my brain simply didn't work in disarray? I decided we needed spreadsheets, or, at least, my mind did.

But, neither Vivian nor I knew how to do spreadsheets. And I was the only one in the office with a Mac computer, so I could communicate with no one. The dean told me that the former person who'd held the position had wanted a Mac and, after she left, they'd not had the budget to replace it. And there still wasn't any money. So my idea for spreadsheets got put on my "to do" list.

Then I became aware of something else I'd taken for granted. In my previous positions, student progression policies had been enforced with little or no wiggle room. If students didn't meet course requirements, they didn't progress to the next semester. Now I found there were policies that looked good on paper, but there had been more wiggle room in enforcing them. I realized this was a bigger system than I'd worked in before, so I thought maybe the largeness made things harder to enforce. But I heard much faculty unrest about this inconsistency. So the progression committee and I took on a Herculean task of revising and organizing the policies to make them clearer and more enforceable. The work of that committee could be a book in itself; their investment, their detailed work, their willing spirit was gargantuan.

Meanwhile, I encountered other faculty concerns, often about perceived inconsistencies in teaching assignments. As faculty members zipped in and out of my office, I kept adding things to my "to do" list so I could follow up.

I found myself rearranging my office a lot. Long before feng shui hit the States, I knew I needed my furniture a certain way to feel comfortable. Vivian laughed. "Every day, Lois, I never know where you'll be sitting." I think now that my "moving behavior" might have been my way of ensuring a calm, orderly place for myself, so I could deal better with my non-stop lists of things to do. Consumed by my lists, I had little awareness of university-wide changes that I learned later were affecting my position.

At the end of each day, after staff and most faculty had gone home, I relished the quiet time while I listened to the day's accumulation of voice mails. Jotting down the caller's initials and a brief note, I soon discovered that each one of the over forty people in the department had different initials. When I figured this out, I chuckled to myself—if this little organizational detail turned me on at the end of a day, I was in the right place.

Once or twice a week, the faculty member who had served as "interim" before me, dropped by with frozen yogurt from the cafeteria: "I know you didn't have time for lunch today."

I'd devour her kind offering.

By fall of my second year, I was intent on getting the schedules on spreadsheet. Pat, the graduate assistant dean, and I had decided to phase in Quattro Pro as monies became available. I still had my Mac computer, so I decided I had to improvise. Marv agreed I should buy my own copy of Quattro Pro for use at home. He loaded it onto the computer we shared, and I stayed up late teaching myself. As I plunked my fingers on the keyboard, I thought a few choice words— I'd never be able to say them aloud—while I hoped the budget would soon allow me to have a computer that was compatible with Mitzi's, my new secretary. Vivian had transferred to another department. A few weeks later, after the program had been loaded on Mitzi's computer, I taught her. Sitting at her keyboard, we made a game of it, acting almost like giggly sisters, blonde and sometimes overwhelmed.

First, we converted the schedules for clinical agency requests. The school used ten different agencies. There were around thirty-five clinical sections (approximately 300 students divided into groups of eight) going to these agencies at different times on different days. When Mitzi finished typing the spreadsheet, we celebrated with high fives. We could locate, with a blink, where any group would be on any day at any time. And I had a clear readable grid to use as I dealt with our agency contracts. I buried old copies of the colorful "kindergarten artwork" in the bottom drawer of my credenza—for the archives. Future generations could get a kick out of our pre-computer primitiveness.

We then put the courses we offered and the faculty teaching assignments on spreadsheets. I was surprised by the responses. When I delivered the course schedule to the registrar, she flopped herself across the counter and hugged me. "I can read them, finally," she said. "Thank you. Thank you. Thank you." When we finished the faculty teaching assignments, I was ready to post them when I found out assignments had never been posted by faculty name rather than by course. I couldn't understand why not; I'd taken that disclosure for granted. I don't remember how the spreadsheet got posted in a faculty conference room, but maybe I got pushy. I do remember faculty gathering to see the listing of what each person was teaching and hearing their muted discussion through the wall to my office next door.

Mitzi and I were proud of the new schedules we'd created. My head was supremely happy with their clarity. Spread out on my conference desk, they would have made chic, black and white, geometric designer wallpaper for the most discerning shopper.

I continued attacking and scratching off items on my "to do" list. Some were minor—organizing contents in the student folders to save time retrieving information, initiating my sitting at registration to troubleshoot student questions, and cutting down the number of my meetings with the four division directors who reported to me when I saw we didn't need them.

Some of my actions, however, seemed to rile up the status quo—starting a separate faculty meeting for my undergraduate faculty (the graduate faculty had their own), supporting the start of open teaching assignment (workload) meetings where faculty could hear the administrative concerns and put in requests, and questioning blurry lines of communication among all of us.

I began to realize that communication was my biggest challenge. My prior experience in smaller settings hadn't prepared me for all the "informal" lines of communication. I often had the feeling: "Who's on first? What's on second?"

When the entire faculty named communication as a concern at a special meeting, I was relieved. The leader had asked us to draw a picture of how we saw communication within nursing. I sketched the straight lines of the formal organizational chart: the dean talks to the assistant deans, the assistant deans to the faculty…. A faculty member sitting next to me squiggled one line randomly all over the page. I glanced over and saw what looked like drizzled chocolate syrup on a plate. She saw me looking and said, "Chaos."

No wonder I'd been confused. Ginny was drawing what was; I was drawing what I'd been accustomed to and what I'd expected it to be. I leaned over and laughed. "No wonder I sometimes feel like I'm the newcomer to outer space."

She said, "I wanted to tell you when you interviewed for the position, Lois. But…"

She didn't finish. But that one statement explained the eerie feeling I'd picked up that day. I know it would not have made a difference though. I've never been one to say no to new experiences and have enjoyed learning to work in new systems.

I continued to have to do my computer work at home every evening; I worked late to finish memos, letters, and documents that I brought to Mitzi on a floppy disc in the morning. Then I was too wired to sleep, so I left voice mails of things I normally would have told faculty the next day. My division directors, especially, teased me about my 2:00 a.m. messages. My frustration grew. What was wrong? Was I menopausal? Was I simply tired? Or was I getting stressed out from the fluid lines of communication that left me feeling confused? I didn't know and started wondering whether I should stay. My second year faculty evaluation was due before Christmas, so I thought I'd wait to see how that turned out before I made a decision. I was happily surprised, but puzzled, when I got what seemed to me inordinately positive ratings on items I took as givens—things that concerned being fair, consistent, and available.

I was granted a third year appointment.

For a short while, I was lulled into thinking I would stay. But then, in January, I had a routine doctor's appointment. The older soft-spoken man sat at his desk, and I sat alongside. He took my blood pressure on my left arm. "Um-m-m. It's off the charts." He announced an absurdly high number.

Bursting into tears, I blurted, "Wha-a-t? My blood pressure is never that high."

He patted my arm. "Must be a bad hair day."

Driving back to work, I knew the "bad hair" was my work. I was running late for a committee meeting and had no time to think. When I entered the room, the five or six faculty members began singing "Happy Birthday." They had prepared a surprise fifty-third birthday party for me—balloons, cake, a game. I choked up. The faculty were consistently supportive. How could I feel so conflicted about staying?

My blood pressure prompted a serious assessment of whether I should stay. I'd cleaned up policies, schedules, and everything else that had come my way. The next year would probably have less clean up and more maintenance. Though it was stressful at times, I had thrived on the clean up part. I had made the difference I'd hoped I could and wasn't sure I'd be content with primarily maintenance activities.

After soul searching, I resigned effective at the end of the semester. It had been one year since Colette had named me Sister Mary Holy Water.

My memory is blurry about that spring. Starting in February, I took a long weekend every other week to visit my dad, who lay dying from bone cancer in Grand Rapids. The week before he passed away, I called him about the birth of our second grandchild, Kyle Jon. My dad's last words to me were, "Blessings on your family." I remember faculty dropping into my office with a word of comfort or a request: "Could you guest lecture again on sexual dysfunction?" "I had my meeting with admissions. Want to hear the stats?" "I've got a problem with a student. Do you have time now?"

Yes, yes, and yes.

My old tape was running; I was ready to leave administration again for teaching. Several faculty encouraged me to apply for a nearby dean position. "You've proven yourself here. That's the next step. Go for it."

But I had no interest. I missed the fun, once again, of working with students. I had another year on my contract. I'd made good friends and chose to stay on to teach. Pat offered me a small office down the hall and promoted one of my division directors to my position. I oriented her and wished her well. And meant it.

When I came back for fall semester a few weeks later, she was working at a new computer. The Mac was gone. I'd emphasized the need for the new one in my end-of-year annual report. I felt my face light up when I saw it. I was thrilled for her; it would make her work much easier. And I was thrilled for me; I could pop my head in and say "Hi, how are you?" and skip along down the hall to my new home among the faculty and near the classrooms.

I loved my new office, a cocoon that held only a desk, a student chair next to it, and a bookcase behind me. A cocoon devoid of dozens of voice mails and visitors. A cocoon of quiet.

Twenty-two

SADIE TOMCZYK

*P*ro and con list. I needed one to consider what I wanted for my next job. Having a warm cozy office was number one for pros. Having to get in and out of my car, year-round, was number one for cons. I couldn't be a home care nurse like Marianna, who loved finding her clients' homes in strange neighborhoods, even taking a broom along in her car to wipe off snow from street signs in order to read them. I shivered when I heard her stories.

It struck me as strange that having an office was important. I never thought of having one when I became a nurse; then being able to run up and down hospital hallways saving lives and feeling important was priority.

The first office I ever had was the one at the general hospital, right after I got my master's degree, when I took the job of nursing education coordinator. The one where the broken crucifix had hung above my desk. It was actually only a cubicle; half walls separated three of us in the same darkish basement room, but it was my own, where I could sit in my new Evan Picone suit.

That was fourteen years ago. Now, the fall of 1995, I had a window view that brought in the morning sun as I sat there in a former assistant dean suit, a deep olive Jones New York, and pondered how to make that year count. I looked forward to my teaching assignments, especially because I'd been able to hand pick them the spring before. Seeking a challenge, I'd assigned myself, along with Jill, a colleague from psychiatric nursing, a few sections of a problematic seminar course. In that course, students did not understand, yet, that seminars were not lecture courses. They wrote scathing evaluations saying they didn't pay the high tuition to hear their fellow students talk. And, in turn, the faculty had unloaded their frustrations on me.

I was certain I could turn the seminar course around; I was immediately deflated. Students, all female—different ages, sizes, and color—sat around a rectangular table: six on each side, three at the far end, me at the head. No one talked, no matter what I did to explain how seminars worked. They hadn't read the assignment before class and nothing I said was going to change that. One student sitting in the middle at the far end wore a baseball cap with the visor down covering her eyes. She was my first student ever to wear a cap to class, and I could never tell if she was sleeping.

As I stumbled through each two-hour session, I examined my reasons for assigning myself to this course. What had made me think I'd have more success than my faculty? I couldn't wait for class to end. I wanted students to slam their unread books into their backpacks and flee. But, no, a tight cluster of three or more stayed after every class to continue the inquisition: "How come you don't lecture? For all we know, you don't even know this stuff. What do you think we're paying for anyway?"

I clearly wasn't God's gift to teaching that I thought I'd be after all my years of encountering a wide array of classroom situations.

At semester's end, Jill, equally attacked, and I evaluated the course and designed a strategy to help the students understand that learning could happen without a lecture, but with more student involvement. We assigned points for all student participation: attending class, bringing in a typed one-page response paper to the readings, and discussing their paper in class. If students earned all their points, they got an A. They could even miss one day of the fifteen sessions and get an A.

I felt smug with the plan; it was sort of like implementing in the classroom the behavior modification techniques that we often saw used on adolescent psychiatric units. You behave well, you get rewarded. If not, you pay the consequences.

During the spring semester, the grading scheme surpassed our expectations. Students seemed to love knowing exactly what was expected of them and the prospect of an attainable A. After class, I found myself loving to hang around to talk. The challenging questions had stopped. I had to remind myself that there is no such thing as an impossible student situation, that it's likely I hadn't figured out how to meet the students' needs. It was the exact same principle I'd taught students from the beginning about how to think about the patient in the hospital bed who has the reputation of "laying on the call bell." "If a patient repeatedly is calling for the nurse," I'd say, "they have an unmet need, and, rather than you unprofessionally complaining about them, it is your job to figure out what that need is and meet it." So if my students were repeatedly complaining about a course, the course wasn't meeting their needs, and I had to figure out how to change it.

I'd also assigned myself to teach a psychiatric clinical. We'd needed another agency to accommodate our numbers of students, and I initiated getting a contract with a hospital where I'd worked med-surg in the early seventies. I had good memories and looked forward to going back there, my eighth place to teach a psych clinical. On my first day back, while I was parked on the street waiting for students to arrive, I recalled working part-time on a thirty-six-bed ward when Jon and Kathleen were preschoolers. I remembered the buzz and excitement of passing hundreds of meds—still arrayed in lineups on aluminum trays, changing smelly soggy dressings on patients having massive disfiguring abdominal and rectal surgeries, and monitoring a dozen or more IVs each PM shift. One of the PM supervisors asked me once why I never punched out until 1:00 a.m. when I should've gotten off at 11:30. I told her I didn't get finished giving my bedtime meds until report time at eleven, so I had to sign off all my charts and meds after I gave report. She was impressed. "Others get off at 11:30. They sign off *before* giving their meds, a no-no as you know. You must have been trained right. Take all the overtime you need; you need not call for approval. When I see your punch card, I'll automatically approve it."

That was not the first time I'd had positive feedback on what I'd been taught at Blodgett. Even though having enough time to get my work finished was frequently a problem, I knew never to compromise the basic principles of what I'd been taught. And, what if, for example, I'd charted on a patient: "Good PM. Up and about. No complaints," before I started giving my nine o'clocks and then found him dead in bed at 10:30? The cross-outs in the chart would be a dead giveaway to the no-no of charting beforehand.

Now I was thankful I could remember that era positively and not have to do that much running around any more. Many nurses my age, fifty-three, were still jogging hospital hallways. The work is tiring. Several had told me over the years that I was lucky I'd been able to go back to school so I could teach. They saw teaching as easier. And they were right, physically, with teaching psychiatric nursing. I didn't have to run anymore for eight hours as they had to do. I could generally saunter or sit, and my clinical teaching shift was usually six hours. I had weekends off. And I'd learned at VU how not to get bored when I'd had to squeeze in all those med reviews with the students.

I came to that clinical relaxed and happy to be there. The staff invited us to participate in all unit activities, a gesture that always made me happy for the students. They'd have access to multiple experiences in which they could observe behaviors and practice therapeutic communication skills.

We were off to a good start. I thought I'd seen most everything in psych clinicals and would sort of coast. For awhile, I did. Early on, we met another "Jesus Christ," reminding me of my very first day of teaching in 1978 at Prairie State College. I remembered how frightened I'd been when a "Jesus Christ" had planted a kiss on my forehead and how I'd had to bluff being calm with my students.

This time, I was not frightened, but tremendously saddened. We had just walked into an adult locked unit when we heard a patient shouting, "I'm Jesus Christ. Get me out of here."

My eight students hovered close behind me as I approached the half-door of the nurses' station directly opposite the patient's room. We could see a young man with long reddish hair and deep-set eyes sitting up in bed and thrashing against the leather restraints around his wrists and ankles. His hairy chest peeked above his patient gown that had fallen down from his arm movement. His face looked like the pictures of Jesus in my childhood story Bible.

Seeing the shock on my students' faces, the charge nurse said, "College student. Ecstasy, one or two doses." A designer drug classified as a hallucinogenic stimulant. "His doctor predicts permanent brain damage."

I could see color drain from my students' faces. One whispered, "This is like that drug commercial that shows frying a brain like an egg."

The patient's mother came to visit. "Jesus Christ" continued to shout and thrash, showing no recognition for her. Students found excuses to stroll past the room, observing the mother's tears as her son hollered at her from his own world.

The post-conference that day was in a blue funk as students talked of the pain that abuse of drugs can cause families. One student said, "I think every one of our classmates should see a person like this. They wouldn't believe it. They'd sure never think of taking drugs again."

She was right. What would it take for young people not to experiment? Should a field trip to a psych unit be mandatory for every teen? Would seeing the effects of drugs stop the behavior?

My coasting along in this clinical hit an emotional breakthrough second semester. One rainy spring morning, a student caught me in the corridor. "Dr.

Roelofs, I can't get my patient to get off the toilet. I need her to go to the dining room for breakfast."

"What's her name?" I asked. As usual, I'd let the students choose their own patients.

"Sadie Tomczyk."

After knocking, I inched into the bathroom with the student and observed an older heavy-set woman bent forward so that I could see only the top of her head. Long stringy grayish hair hung over her face.

"Sadie," I said, standing alongside her. "My name is Lois Roelofs, and I am your nursing student's teacher. Amy wants to take you to breakfast."

"I'm not finished yet. And, I'm not hungry," Sadie said, in a low, loud staccato monotone.

I'd heard this voice before. Where? When? I looked up to think. Surprise surged through my shoulders. She was the Sadie I had had in my therapy group when I was a graduate student sixteen years earlier. The Sadie who gave me the idea of studying the leisure preferences of nursing home residents for my master's thesis. The Sadie who gave me the plastic red rose in the egg-shaped vase.

I had not remembered her last name. She was simply Sadie to me, a very special Sadie.

"I think we've met before, Sadie." The overwhelming coincidence made it difficult to speak.

"I know we have," Sadie spit out, never looking up. "Don't you remember I told you about having epilepsy? I told you how my family put me away?"

Amy looked at me over Sadie's head as if to say, "What's going on here?"

"Yes, I do remember, Sadie," I said, steadying my voice. "My classmate Janice and I met you in group about sixteen years ago when you lived at Wilmington Gardens. I still have the rose you gave me as a present. It's on my desk at work. I've never forgotten you."

I still couldn't see Sadie's face. Her short, straight, dark bob of sixteen years earlier had changed to long, lifeless graying strands. Her bright housedresses, colored socks, and white laced heels had faded to her wrinkled patient gown, pale bare legs, and nonskid, blue patient slippers.

"I'm finished now. I'll go to breakfast," Sadie said, resuming her staccato monotone, still looking at the floor.

Amy and I assisted the hunched old woman to stand, and then we pivoted her smelly, sluggish body into her wheelchair. Empathy wrote itself into Amy's face as she was beginning to grasp the situation.

I wandered to the nurses' station, stunned. Memories washed through me. While Sadie had been shuttled among psychiatric facilities, she'd been my inspiration for both my master's and doctoral research on leisure. While she'd been confined to institutional living, I'd moved once, raised a family, earned two advanced degrees, and moved up the career ladder to administrative positions. While she'd been restricted to life with caregivers, I'd been free to live among family, friends, neighbors, students, and colleagues.

I wanted to weep. I wanted to hug her. I wanted to tell her, "I'm sorry for how your illness has limited your life." Remembering my own hospitalization behind locked doors nearly thirty years earlier, I shuddered thinking her circumstances could've been mine.

I got the keys to the unit bathroom out of the drawer. In front of the unbreakable mirror found on psychiatric units, I stared at myself, searching my eyes, for a long time. Grabbing onto the sink, I prayed, *Thank you, God, for all the things I take for granted. My health, my husband, my kids, my grandkids.*

The next day, I brought in my eighty-page, bound master's thesis to show my students and the staff the opening quote, Sadie's words: "What do they expect me to do? Sit outside and smell the car exhaust?" Standing in the nurses' station, I told them the story of how Sadie's frustration had been the impetus for my leisure preference study sixteen years earlier. As the reality and longevity of Sadie's illness seeped into each person's heart, a funeral-like silence blanketed the nurses' station.

I reminded the students, just like our experience with the college student who had taken Ecstasy, that the best way to learn psychiatric nursing is to have personal connections with people who are experiencing a mental illness. They teach us that they're human. They remind us that each person counts. They teach us to care.

PART FIVE

Tenure

Twenty-three

GOING BACK

ois, this is Christina Thorsen at Trinity…I'm wondering if I could interest you in coming back. Our full-time mental health position is open."

Christina—she'd started as the chair of Trinity's nursing department the same year I'd started as assistant dean at Xav's. We'd met, briefly, at a few professional meetings.

"And, I'd like you to teach nursing research. And to help out again in ortho clinicals." Christina spoke softly with a feeling of urgency.

Sitting in my cozy cocoon office at Xav's listening to Christina's voice, I suddenly felt warm all over. My love for Trinity had never left. I'd been gone five years. Holding four different positions in three places during that time felt like I'd taken a self-imposed sabbatical for renewal—trying research and teaching and administrative positions in larger, university settings. And succeeded. Was that what God had intended? Unlike people who always know God's call, I never knew for sure. I identified more with Marianna's, "Trust your gut." But, then, come to think of it, God was probably talking to me through my gut. But not in the clear words from above I would've appreciated.

I had a feeling, yet, that with my doctorate I should try to teach at the master's and doctoral level. I consulted with my brother, Dewey, a Harvard-educated philosopher teaching undergraduates. He assured me I could be fulfilled teaching at that level, even though I'd been socialized in my doctoral program to think of teaching in higher education. "You'll have more time for your own scholarly work if you don't have to serve on thesis committees of master's or doctoral students," he said. "And you'll have more time to enjoy your students if you don't have the stringent 'publish or perish' tenure requirements of a Big Ten university."

He affirmed what I knew to be true.

A few weeks later, spring 1996, I stood in my old lecture room giving a faculty presentation for consideration for rehire. I compared nursing theories and preached about the merits of theory-based nursing education and practice. Preparing for the presentation, I realized how much I'd missed this kind of intellectual rigor while I was administrative. I thought of the detour I'd taken since my doctoral research, how I hadn't followed through with presentations and publications.

I needed to honor Sadie and get the message out about how mental illness and aging can limit choices in leisure time. And can limit choices in life. I needed to speak for her.

Sensing receptive faces in the audience, I knew it was time for me to go back. It was time for me to realize, once and for all, I liked working with people more than paper—that working with students was infinitely more fun than being immersed in memos, annual reports, and minutes of meetings. And, at fifty-four, I wanted a place where I could enjoy the final stage of my career, the eight years until Social Security kicked in or possibly the eleven years until retirement age.

After the lecture, I met with representatives of the Board of Trustees and my former academic dean. One asked: "Lois, you left once before. What assurance do we have that you won't leave again?"

"None." I answered, flippantly. "Keep me challenged." And I meant that; I could not imagine being stuck teaching the same courses or doing the same things forever.

I would be going back to Trinity with a renewed commitment to teaching. In the past year alone, I'd learned that any yen for administration had disappeared from my bones. I'd learned I could fail wretchedly teaching a new course, and then make it successful. I'd learned from meeting another "Jesus Christ," but especially from meeting Sadie again, that I needed to return to my mission of teaching others to care about those having mental illness.

The evening after the interview, Marv said, "I suppose you'll want help moving again. I think I still have the boxes in the attic."

I would be moving into a new office; the nursing department at Trinity had moved to another building since I'd left. I could feel the excitement returning. That fall I was not disappointed. I loved my new office—Trinity's grassy quad out the window, pale gray walls, soft blue carpeting, light oak furniture. The promising smell of newness. To the left of my desk, a "student chair," waiting to be occupied. A former friend and colleague's office on one side, Christina's on the other. The secretary in the outer office attracting a stream of pitter-patter, chitchat, and laughter.

Twenty-four

THINGS I TRIED

As students sauntered into the classroom, their burning glances melted my smile. Even though it was my first time to teach nursing research, I'd wanted the challenge and I was ready. Or thought I was. I'd prepared the syllabus, planned the assignments, and written my first few lectures. But I had heard the course had a reputation. Students knew before they came that they were going to hate it.

In the past, some had successfully petitioned to take an easier course off campus during the summer. This year Dr. Thorsen had denied permission. They were stuck with me, the new—recycled, I called myself—teacher in Trinity's nursing program.

I remembered hating my own undergraduate course in research, but thought since I had loved my research experiences as a master's and doctoral student I could make the course absolutely scintillating for the students. And I thought with my enthusiasm that I would effortlessly be able to change their attitudes. I could chatter about how they could design research studies, collect data, analyze the data, and present their findings—in effect, change the world of nursing practice with their marvelous findings.

I wasn't prepared for my inability to kindle the fire. Or even bring the matchsticks. Over the next four years, I would teach the course five times. And I would try anything, everything, in those five times to motivate that burning for learning that I'd had myself.

I tried joking. "What an honor it is for me to teach the most hated course in the nursing program. Think of it! Not everyone gets this chance."

They pasted sullen stares on their faces. Had I been here before? Visions of me singing the Oscar Meyer wiener song flew into my mind.

I tried more humor. "I love this course, and I never want to hear you say you don't. I don't care what you say to others, but, to me, you must say you love it. And, who knows, if you keep repeating this, it may turn out to be true."

They launched "you've got to be crazy" looks.

I tried having students do a mock presentation. "Today, I've brought one of my research papers with corresponding slides of the findings. Each of you can take a turn and come up front to read a section of the paper with the accompanying slides. You can pretend you're presenting at a conference being held in a Hyatt Regency ballroom."

They complied, most without emotion, and, when they came forward from their seat, each tripped over the extension cord for the slide projector.

How could they not be excited about this? I was jubilant merely thinking of the possibilities for them. I tried telling them about the time when my poster presentation won First Place in the doctoral student category at the Midwest Nursing Research Society conference at the Hyatt Regency right here in Chicago. Me, at fifty, ancient next to most of my classmates. How, at the time, I almost missed the announcement because I was having a cup of coffee with an old friend and was going to skip the business meeting where awards were announced. I wanted to impress upon my students that if I, a former suburban housewife and mom, could become a successful researcher, they could surely become one too.

I think I overdid it sometimes. One student's evaluation warned me to quit bragging about myself. But, who knows? For sure, I succeeded with another who said I was "full of fire" for this subject and my fire "helped a lot." Whenever I got end-of-semester student evaluations, I always remembered my very first evaluation in 1981 as a nursing education coordinator. During an orientation of nursing students to our hospital, I'd presented what I thought was an animated, organized, and interesting vision of the hospital's mission statement for 100 students. Ninety-nine said I did a fantastic job; one said the time spent on the mission statement was a waste of time. I never forgot that one.

I tried asking one class to be my research subjects. Attitudes were brighter that semester, and students readily agreed. Since I knew of their church affiliations, I designed a study to answer this question: Why, from your own religious background, should you as a nursing student study nursing research?

Using this study, I showed students how I analyzed their written responses, using the same procedures I'd done with the over 1,000 pages of data I'd gathered from my own interviews for my doctoral dissertation. How I read their responses line by line to identify codes (words and phrases), and then clustered similar codes under six broader themes. For example, for the theme "Following God's Mandate" a student had written: "As Christians we have an obligation to use our minds the best we can, and we are to promote good." For "Gaining Wisdom," "God has created this universe with many questions, some of which may be answered. Research helps us to comprehend and utilize various findings." And the theme of "Assuring Quality" emerged from this response: "We as Christians should promote advancement of healthcare and caring for patients…always keeping in mind what is good for the patient."

They were as pleased with these results as I was. I even submitted an abstract and presented these findings at a national conference. Other undergraduate nursing faculty teaching research thought the variable of the student's religious beliefs to be an innovative and helpful way to engage the student in this course, a problem many of them also had.

Once, I tried a new approach to students' complaints about an exam. I asked to see each one individually so I could listen and take notes about what was problematic for them. I grouped their responses into seven categories and offered solutions. For example, for the problem of *erasing* answers on the Scantron sheet and having the scanner misread them: "Ensure you have a super-duper eraser and you do super-duper erasing." For *glazing*—when eyes go into a stare from feeling overwhelmed from terminology: "Take mini breaks…. Sing a song (to yourself, not out loud)…." For *tiring* during the exam: "Give your head a break. Follow glazing solution."

I shared these results of my new theory I called "Bombing Answers" with the students. One said, "You can design a study out of anything!" I said, "That's the point. You have a problem, any problem, bugging you in practice? Study it!"

A few courses later, when I thought my challenging days were over, I handed back a first test and read a few faces of contempt among the class of about fifteen students. A student to my left raised her hand and asked with an edge to her voice, "How were we supposed to know the answers? I read all the assigned readings and I studied my notes, but none of it was on the test."

I tried agreeing. "You're right," I said. "The test was not a spit-back facts kind of test. It wasn't enough to know fact A and fact B. You needed to figure out, together, fact A and fact B would give you C, and that would be the answer. You needed to use your critical thinking skills."

A hand shot up on the right side of the classroom. With eyes ablaze, another student asked, "What do you mean 'critical thinking'?"

I explained.

She retorted, "I thought this was a research course. If I'd known it was a critical thinking course, I wouldn't have taken it."

I tried humor again. Covering my ears with my hands and frowning in mock horror, I cried, "Oh, oh, oh. I'm going to pretend I didn't hear that. Dr. Thorsen would have a heart attack." It dawned on me, instantly, we, as a faculty, might have lofty goals of teaching students to think critically, but there was no module in the curriculum specifically teaching the process.

I tried agreeing, but also accepting responsibility. "You are so right! We know it's in your student handbook, but if you don't know what it means, then we as a faculty have not done our job."

Tension defused. Share ownership for the problem, I reminded myself. The next class we discussed a handout I'd made on critical thinking. And I was thankful the other courses I was teaching were going smoothly.

Soon after the "critical thinking" episode, I did a mini-survey to see how the class was going. One student wrote, "The best thing I like about this class is your dress." I shared the results with the class, and we all laughed.

Humor helped.

I tried changing textbooks. From a super-duper, high-level, densely written, wonderfully informative text, to a user-friendly book with just the basic information and an accompanying workbook. The only good thing about this change was that students, who never read a word in the heavy-duty book, now had to read to help their group members fill out the worksheets in class.

I tried matching my wardrobe to the lecture. For ethnography, the study of people in other cultures, I wore Mardi Gras beads and a pink straw sombrero, For phenomenology, the study of a person's lived experience, I carried a catheter bag; people needing permanent indwelling urinary catheters would have specific characteristics that would help define how they lived. For grounded theory—the methodology I'd used in my doctoral research on leisure—I wore a beige crocheted beach dress over my taupe tencel Nordstrom jumper to show how a theory could be generated by interviewing subjects about their leisure time. They heard even more about the theory I'd generated that I'd named "Authoring Leisure."

I even tried taking them to local research conferences. There they learned what a keynote speaker was, and that other people besides me presented posters and oral presentations. They sat attentively and looked like professionals; some even attended one session I presented. I was proud of them.

But I was most proud when a friend, a dean at a larger college of nursing, invited my students to present the research posters they'd made, depicting existing studies, alongside the students at her college. I drilled my students on professional presentation: what to wear (dark slacks, white top), what information to put on their note cards, and how to time their presentation. As I made rounds among them after their presentations, they confided how spiffy they felt next to many of the other school's students who were wearing jeans and who had rambled over the time limit. When their faculty came up to me one by one to compliment me on the professionalism of my students, I, of course, lit up like the world's largest bonfire.

In passing along the compliments to my students, their eyes sparkled, too, and I knew there'd be researchers among them in the future. And that my enthusiasm would be remembered, at least by some. On the way home after dark, I tried not to split the kick pleat of my suit skirt as I hip-hopped in my navy pumps through dirty, snowy slush in a Baskin-Robbins parking lot to celebrate with a double-dip, butter-pecan sugar cone. Settling back into my car, I felt myself suddenly poop out, weary with worry about my personal life.

Twenty-five

STORMS OF ILLNESS

ou need my massage therapist!" Joanie, the self-proclaimed "energizer bunny" and marathon runner of our nursing faculty said. "Peter will cure whatever ails you!"

"Peter?" I wasn't sure I heard correctly.

"Yes, he's an older man, a family friend. He gives my referrals a special rate."

I'd invited a few of my colleagues for lunch—chicken salad and zucchini bread. I'd been to Seattle that summer to welcome our third grandchild, Megan Annalynn, and had just taught an August two-week catch-up course for junior transfer students. It was 1997. As I sipped raspberry iced tea, I had said, "I don't know how I'm going to start fall semester. I'm so tired and my muscles burn from head to toe." Joanie had hopped to my rescue.

I'd only had two massages in my life—by females. But I was desperate, and I was cheap.

As I lay nude, wrapped in the warm ambience of flutes and lavender and waterfalls, Peter began to explain, with his hands up high, an inch or two beneath his gray bearded kindly face, what he was going to do. Then, abruptly, he stopped.

"What's wrong?" I asked, ready to jet directly into the clouds.

"I'm feeling a lot of energy. Energy I usually feel only very close to the body."

Energy! I had just taught Martha Rogers' theory of nursing that addressed human beings as energy fields. The students would love this story. I could hear their teasing: "You went to a *man*? You took *all* your clothes off? And you were throwing off *energy*?"

"Have you been unusually busy lately?" he asked.

"Yes, I have." I said, trying to breathe deeply so I wouldn't appear as scared as I felt. "I just finished an intensive teaching stint. Then we took a quick trip to Michigan to see my husband's oldest brother, who's dying from prostate cancer, and now fall semester is starting."

He started the massage, and my mind raced into the semester ahead.

Besides classes and clinicals to teach, I had other responsibilities as a faculty member. I was eligible for promotion and tenure, so I'd just started what would become about a thirty-hour process of writing a self-evaluation and compiling supporting documents.

And stacks of curriculum revision materials stood on my desk. When I'd come back to Trinity the fall before, faculty anointed me with my former position of curriculum chair.

And I was concentrating on my scholarly work—conducting further analysis of my doctoral research, submitting abstracts, preparing poster and paper presentations, flying to conferences.

I was excited about these activities and enjoyed how they broadened my faculty role. I'd never been content with being only a mom, or a nurse, or a teacher. My mind always needed more.

During the two-hour massage, I concentrated on visualizing my twenty-one time blocks available each week, three each day—morning, afternoon, and evening—as I'd often counseled students to do, and as I'd done as a doctoral student, when overwhelmed. I sketched in what I had to do, leaving, as was my habit, mental health time—free time—in the Saturday and Sunday morning slots. By the time the massage was finished, I'd planned my calendar for the semester.

I had not, however, built in time blocks for my personal life to hit troubled waters.

In late September, a few weeks after my energy-jazzed massage, my sister Esther called from Grand Rapids, "Dave has cancer again. Prostate."

Now prostate cancer had hit my family. Besides Marv's oldest brother who was dying, another brother and eight others in his extended family had had prostate cancer.

In October, as I was dealing with follow-up phone calls about Dave, Marianna called from her new home in D.C. Before I could even say hello, she blurted: "I've got cancer."

"No!" I screamed. "For real?" I felt as though I'd been flattened by a bomb.

"For real. Breast," she replied, matter-of-factly.

We had always joked about being nurses who never have a simple symptom without thinking it was cancer. Any pain, any bleeding, any diarrhea—it was probably cancer.

I didn't know what to say. We had shared almost everything over twenty-five years and in less than five seconds I felt like a stranger.

November was a blur of teaching classes and clinicals, dealing with phone calls about cancer treatments, and having massages to dull my now ever-present fatigue and muscle pain.

In early December, Marv's oldest brother died, his six-year struggle with cancer over. The family gathered in Michigan. Our group of nine siblings with nine spouses now numbered seventeen. We lined up for a picture with the first vacant spot. The empty place haunted me.

I returned to the college and met with the Academic Affairs committee of the Board of Trustees once again. I left the meeting having been granted the best there could be—tenure and promotion to Full Professor. I walked back to my office so tired in body and spirit I could barely smile as a colleague grabbed me in a hug with congratulations.

During Christmas vacation, Marianna and I met in Seattle where we were each visiting our children. We sat silently, tear-filled, and sipped mochas on easy chairs by the piano at Nordstrom in Northgate, her experience of cancer now separating us. It was the first time in our long friendship we were actually wordless. Christmas shoppers crowded past with their colorful packages, while the piano player pounded out "Silver Bells."

Early January we buried Aunt Maggie, who died of complications after emergency surgery. The aunt who had welcomed Marv and me into her basement apartment when we had moved to Chicago thirty years earlier. At the funeral luncheon, I said to a cousin, "It's amazing how fast things happen. A week ago she was fine."

A week later, my Michigan sister called to report on a visit with my mother. Mother had said, "Ninety-five would be a good round number to die."

Esther told her, "You have to wait until Saturday. People are coming for your party."

We were due to celebrate our mutual birthdays that weekend in Michigan. Kathleen and I were hoping for snow-free roads. Some years the road conditions kept us home.

Right after my mother's birthday luncheon, my sister Kay and I helped her into bed for a nap. She, still wearing the red polka-dot dress I'd given her, clutched her chest in pain and waved me off to start our drive home. I leaned over her side rail to say, "I love you little."

"I love you big," she replied, weakly, with a vacant look to her weary eyes.

"I love you like…" I waited for her to finish the phrase.

"A little pig," she whispered, with her eyes closed and a slight wave of her hand.

Our life-long *good-bye* ritual. She died forty-eight hours later. I left my office at the college immediately and drove back to Michigan to see her empty room and make funeral plans. Marv and Kathleen would be coming two days later for the funeral. So I could ride back with them in threatening January weather, I called a student living about a half hour away, that I knew was home for the weekend, to see if he knew anyone who could drive my car back. He immediately said, "No problem."

"You're sure?" I hadn't expected the quick response.

"I'm sure. I'll figure it out. I can pick up your car tomorrow morning. Where will it be?"

"At Zaagman's Funeral Home on Eastern. My sister and I will be there making the funeral plans." I was still having a problem thinking he would do this for me. "I'll leave my keys under the mat."

I found out later he and his girlfriend, also a nursing student, had driven into Grand Rapids to pick up my car. Instead of driving back to school together, one of them drove my car. The next day, after the funeral, there was a snowstorm on the way home around Benton Harbor. I was thankful to be safely in the backseat peeking at the whiteout between the tall floral arrangements flanking my sides. Kathleen kept Marv alert with her chatter. When we got home, tears came when Marv pressed the garage door opener and I saw our headlights light up the taillights of my car safely tucked into the garage. I was relieved to know the generous person who had driven it home for me was safely back, too.

The day after the funeral, I taught three hours straight. I'd lost time and needed to introduce my mental health nursing course and include the first lecture as well. Wanting the students to have a positive experience, I acted as if nothing had happened except my mother had died. "She wanted to die," I said, "because my dad died four years ago, and she missed him. So her death was a *blessing*."

I thought I'd convinced myself.

In May, at the end of the semester, I drove to Michigan to visit the cemetery, Rest Lawn. I bought a mocha a half mile away and settled down on the grass in the sun close to my parents' graves. A woman stood nearby and asked who I was there for. I pointed, "For my folks, over there, Dewey and Theresa—Tess—Hoitenga."

She walked away, and my grieving erupted. I ran to my car, closed the windows in the May heat, and covered my drenched face in a hankie. I started calling people on my car phone. The first to answer was my sister Rose in Seattle.

"What on earth is wrong?" she asked.

"The folks are dead, Rose," I sobbed.

Forty-five minutes later, sobbed dry, I bought an assortment of cut flowers at the gardening store next to the cemetery, poked a Rest Lawn container in the ground above my mother's name, and said out loud, "Sorry, Mother, I lack your skillful symmetry in floral arranging." I imagined her striking blue eyes twinkling. I drove on a few miles to Marv's sister Linda who met me at her kitchen door. She took in my most certainly stricken face and opened her arms to envelop me as I broke into more sobs.

Summer that year was a time for healing—no more life-changing phone calls. We had one small scare. Returning from a business trip downstate, Marv said, "What could be wrong if it feels like a vise-like pain when I'm sitting too long in the car?"

I didn't know. But he'd also been having fatigue—unusual for his Type A personality—and urinary frequency during the night, breaking his life-long pattern of sleeping from nine to four. With my insistence, he saw a doctor and was diagnosed with prostatitis and started antibiotic treatment. His PSA was 1.1, well below the danger zone of 4. We were relieved.

The fall of 1998 started with a shocking phone call late one Sunday evening from Marv's sister Linda in Grand Rapids. "There's been a terrible accident. Shirley's [another sister] okay. She was thrown from the pickup and needed a hundred stitches. But Harm's quadriplegic. He's got a five percent chance to live." I stood by the phone, stunned.

I typed a letter informing my students about my brother-in-law and dropped it off at the college before seven the next morning. Marv and I drove three somber hours to the ICU. Standing at Harm's bedside, I recalled my early nursing experience on the night shift with a teen-aged patient. Danny was paralyzed from the neck down in a diving accident. Sitting on a footstool, I listened to his dashed dreams—no more cars, girls, football, or college. While he lay on his stomach on a circle bed, I looked into his eyes, dabbed his tears, positioned his straw, wiped his mouth.

As I observed Harm's unresponsive body invaded by tubes and wires and immobilizing devices, I turned to one of my nieces, "Have you thought about a 'Do Not Resuscitate' order?"

"Don't even go there, Aunt Lois," she said. It was clear the three daughters had discussed this and were set on helping their folks fight.

At the end of the day, Marv wheeled his sister Shirley, with her IV stand, from her room to the ICU to see Harm for the first time since the accident the day before. She stood, carefully, to lean over the side rail. "Hon, I'm here," she said, in her soft kindly voice, tears forming.

From his comatose state, Harm's eyes fluttered open, and he directed them, for a split second, toward Shirl's voice. Tears dropped all around the bed. We grabbed each other's hands while a chaplain prayed, "Please restore this man, oh Lord, if it be thy will."

Back on the highway, I sobbed all the way to Kalamazoo, forty-five minutes away. "Honey, they don't know. They simply don't know what's in store for them should he live."

I felt as if my insides were grating over a grid of sharp steel spikes.

A few weeks after the accident, my husband's family gathered in Minnesota, this time to bury another sister's husband after an eleven-month cancer illness. Talking in hushed tones, we shared news of Harm's struggle for life. When everyone left for the funeral home, I sat alone at my sister-in-law's kitchen table and began to cry and pray, *No more, God, please no more.*

Now there were only sixteen of the original eighteen for the family picture.

We hurried ten hours home across Wisconsin to Chicago and resumed speeding lives.

A few days later, during a ten-minute break between classes, I rushed to my computer to get a progress report on my sister Rose's husband in Seattle who was having open-heart surgery. "He's losing blood. He may not live."

I rushed back to the classroom—stoic teacher that I was—and began to explain a video. Then I broke down in tears for the first time in my twenty years of teaching. I quickly started the video and ran for my office. Our secretary saw me, and without my asking, called Christina, my department chair, out of her office to see if she could take over the class. Gratefully, I threw stuff into my briefcase, flew past the open door of the classroom, drove home in a fog, fell into bed, and cried more.

That fall I was honored to make my first site visit as a nursing program evaluator for the American Association of Colleges of Nursing. I spent several weeks preparing to visit a college several states away—reading a stack of materials and beginning a draft of the report. During the three-day, two-night visit, the chair of my team, who served as my mentor, and I compiled and typed our report until four each morning. By surprise, we encountered a campus emerging from a natural disaster and a few deaths. My mentor taught me how to guide the faculty, now grieving, through the dreaded evaluation process. They thanked us over and over after we read our positive report at the end of our visit. Fatigued beyond anything I ever imagined, I choked with emotion as I listened to their generous thank yous.

That same fall, I was also appointed to a national committee on nursing program evaluation and immediately looked forward to its biannual meetings in Washington, D.C. I called Marianna. "Guess what! I'll be coming twice a year! I'll arrange to stay over a day or two. Plan on me in January."

I felt as if I'd reached a peak in my career of being a nursing educator—starting as a clinical instructor and progressing to the classroom; teaching in associate, bachelor, and, master's programs; serving administratively as an acting chair and as an assistant dean; and now, with these background experiences, being able to volunteer as a national site visitor to other nursing programs and as a member of a national committee.

But my life also felt like a raft on white-water rapids. No guide, no paddle, no life vest. Even though the illnesses of our family and friends had improved or stabilized, there was no time to slow down or reflect.

Twenty-six

CANCER

ntibiotics didn't improve Marv's symptoms. An ultrasound and biopsy followed. Four days before Christmas, Kathleen, now twenty-nine and living nearby, stopped over and the three of us were gabbing around the kitchen table. The phone rang. Marv answered. A long silence followed. He hung up, turned to us, and announced with the terror of devastating news in his eyes and voice: "I have cancer."

Speechless, we formed a circle, hugged, and sobbed. My world went black.

Due to Christmas weekend, we had to wait five days for the "options" appointment. Marv asked the urologist about nerve-sparing surgery to prevent impotence. He answered quickly, "That's not my priority. If I have to cut all around to make sure I get the cancer, I don't even attempt to save the nerve."

After pausing a second, he looked first at Marv, then at me, then back to Marv and said, "You've had your children." And, after a pause, as if trying to figure it out, he added, "You don't...you don't still...?"

Don't what? Plan to have more kids at age fifty-six? Make love at our age? Shock set in. Didn't he know this was a couple's disease? That, when the man becomes surgically impotent, both their lives change forever?

He suggested a support group. It was clear he didn't care to know about what we as a family and as an extended family had experienced with PSAs and digital rectal exams, biopsies and surgeries, chemo and radiation, vacuum pumps and penile implants, dying and death.

Where was the caring I expected from health care professionals? The caring I had taught my nursing students for years and years? Not here. Our unasked questions went unacknowledged and unanswered.

The last months of uncertainty had left us shaken. I tried to shove my unresponsive God in a closet. But the door cracked open a few times. Three people—my sister Rose, a friend, and a nursing colleague—called me. They'd seen a urologist from a nearby university hospital on TV explaining nerve-sparing surgery that increased the odds of not becoming impotent. They knew of our family impotency stories and how this might be a fear for Marv. They gave us the name.

In early January, Jon called from Seattle. "Hi, Mom. Sheri and I want to come and see you and Dad while you're waiting for surgery. Sheri's folks will take care of the kids. We'd like to come on your birthday, since it's the first one you'll have without Grandma."

Had it only been a year since my mother died two days after our mutual birthday?

At O'Hare a few weeks later, Marv waited in the car. When I saw Jon and Sheri coming up the escalator to baggage claim, backpacks in place like college kids, I burst into tears.

February 18, 1999. Kathleen and I accompanied Marv to the surgical waiting room of the University of Chicago Hospitals. He left us, face drawn, at ten in the morning. Kathleen reached for my hand as we watched him follow a nurse. Sadness swept through me. I didn't know what to expect from the surgery, and I didn't know this hospital. Strange hallways, strange cafeteria, strange people. We loitered over lunch and haphazardly read magazines I'd packed. The nurse came with her last update for the day at 7:30 that evening. "He's doing fine," she said gently, handing me a hospital-embossed vinyl garment bag of his jeans, crew-neck sweater, and shoes. "We can go to the Oncology Unit now."

Me, on an oncology unit. I thought back to my early days with Prairie State students when I'd had two clinical groups of twelve, each for two days a week, on an oncology unit. I taught students how to bathe terminally ill patients, how to listen to their fears, how to comfort them. But I didn't feel competent now to help my own husband. Or myself.

We stepped off the elevator. A sandy-haired man, thirty-ish, wearing green scrubs and carrying a clipboard padded with papers, was walking toward us. "Hi, Dr. Roelofs, I've assigned myself to your husband."

It was Doug, one of my former Trinity graduates. I flew toward him, squashing him and his clipboard with my hug. Other grads, Aimee and Debbie, also were there, waiting for me with hugs in the center of the hallway. God was watching. How had I dared to doubt?

The pathology report showed the entire tumor had been removed. There'd be no need for chemo or radiation. The crucial nerve had been saved. We were numb with relief and gratitude.

After class one day, an older student lagged behind, "Are you all right, Dr. Roelofs?"

I assured her I was fine, while I marveled at how perceptive she was. I was not fine, and faculty, too, had been asking me. I had assured them I was hanging in, that I was getting the "help" I needed—a euphemism for finding a therapist to help me get my raft to calmer waters. When I'd told the therapist about my personal and family events, over ten in a fifteen-month period, each qualifying for a crisis on any life event scale, I heard, "Sounds like you're bouncing along the bottom." As I mopped up my sopped face with tissues from the ever-present box in therapists' offices, I thought, *Wow, good "therapeutic communication" response!* My students could have done as well. But, indeed, I needed help to get back up to the water's surface.

That summer, we threw a triple-celebration party. Marv had survived surgery, Kathleen had graduated from a master's program, and we had finished an addition onto our house. Jon and Sheri came from Seattle with Kristin, now seven, Kyle, five, and Megan, two. Cars from a hundred friends lined the driveway and the street. It was such a happy day that, after taking pictures of our grandchildren and guests in the back yard, I went out front and took pictures of the filled street to capture the momentary glow I felt around the entire house.

About that time, I read an ad describing a discussion group at Borders on Julia Cameron's *The Artist's Way*. An actress would run the group to help people explore their creativity. I saw the topic and the leader as a fresh perspective on life—far away from nursing. In the class, I learned to unclutter my house and my head to make room for my right brain to emerge.

One day the instructor told us to make a collage: "You have three minutes to tear words and pictures out of these magazines and to glue them onto a sheet of poster paper. Choose pictures that make you think of who you'd like to be. Start now!"

In the middle of my collage, the Viagra couple danced. In the lower right-hand corner, a torn paper fragment read: "Take this job and shove it." What did this mean? I'd never thought to quit my job. Maybe Freud knew.

At the end of the summer, at Marv's forty-year high school reunion in Minnesota, he shared our joke of using Viagra for the first time six weeks after surgery. How we sat in our family room and waited for it to work. How disappointed we were when nothing happened. How it did work while Marv was showering before bed. How, when he presented himself, I said, "Where did you get that?" As if he'd been out shopping. He suggested to folks that it's best if you read the directions before taking the medication. People laughed to tears and, afterwards, thanked us for *being real*. Several shared their hurtful secrets with me that they hadn't been able to tell anyone else. Secrets that couldn't be public. I hurt for everybody. Why must we act as if we've got it all together? Why can't we allow ourselves to be vulnerable? Why must we wear facades?

I could hear myself challenging my nursing students: "What do you think about people not feeling free to talk about mental health concerns? What do you think about them feeling as if they will be judged if they tell their stories? From your upbringing, how do you think these people should be treated?"

The reunion ended past midnight, way past Marv's nine o'clock bedtime. We traded stories as we drove the half-hour to his brother's farm and happily fell into bed in the second-floor bedroom as soon as we got there. As I fell asleep, I heard groaning sounds through the open window coming from the pole barn behind the house. The cattle. Or was it the pigs?

The next morning, one classmate's mother, in her eighties, approached us as we climbed the steps of church. "I hear you were the life of the party last night, Marv. Everyone went home and told their folks." She laughed as she grabbed his arm. "Your story is all over town."

Others greeted us in the foyer with the same news. Many smiles, lots of laughs.

That afternoon, we started home. East on Highway 7 toward Minneapolis. Between fields of corn, beets, and soybeans. I turned the air-conditioner on low.

"I'm glad we went to my reunion," Marv said. "It's clear I livened up the party once again, even though I didn't intend to."

"For sure," I said, "by telling our story. Do you think anything will come of it?"

"Hard to say. It's clear from the response we got at church that we broke some code of silence. Maybe now some people will feel safe enough to tell their stories.... They can use us as an example." The warm rays of the sun shimmered on the car's hood as Marv looked over at me, smiled, and placed his hand over mine. "Hope so."

My mind wandered to worrying about Marv's recuperation. It had been slower than we'd expected. We almost hadn't gone to the reunion. Fatigue remained. Scans had shown abnormal lesions on his liver and lungs. What did they mean? Metastasis? Or were his numerous failed attempts to quit smoking catching up with him? To calm my forever-raging stomach, I repeatedly tried to tell myself Marv would be one of the lucky ones. I had to; I simply couldn't envision the alternative.

Twenty-seven

TRUSTING GOD

*Y*ou may be eligible to apply for a sabbatical," Christina, my department chair, reminded me when we got back after Marv's high school reunion. If I were granted one, I'd be free to deal with whatever happened to Marv health-wise and have time to finish scholarly work my faculty role expected. On November 10, 1999, I submitted the following application to our professional development committee:

> This document constitutes my application for a sabbatical leave for the fall 2000 semester. The purpose for the sabbatical is to complete two projects I have started....
>
> The first project I am proposing to complete for this sabbatical is to publish completed research on the impact of using qualitative research methods on older adults. When I conducted my qualitative/grounded theory method dissertation on older adults' leisure, I added three questions at the end of my interview guide that addressed a) what the experience of the interview was like for them, b) how my presence in their retirement home during a period of participant observation influenced them, and c) why they were willing to participate in my study....
>
> After completion of all dissertation requirements dealing with the central topic of leisure, I analyzed the data (n = 40) from these three questions related to use of qualitative methods. Between 1994 to 1997, I presented the findings at three local and regional research conferences in both paper and poster format. The findings were enthusiastically received by conference participants, and I was encouraged to disseminate them in published form....
>
> ...My timeline for completion would be four to six weeks.

I envisioned nice long days at the computer like I'd spent writing my dissertation. I'd read and type from 8:00 to 12:00 in the morning, then drive a few miles for a double-scoop Hawaiian Delight or butter-pecan ice cream cone at Plush Horse (I figured the calories may be equivalent to a meat and cheese sandwich lunch), then come back home for a 1:00 to 4:00 repeat of the morning. At 4:00, I'd take an hour walk before Marv came home.

The final six to eight weeks I'd work on the next project:

> The second project I am proposing to complete for this sabbatical is to complete the necessary work for a publishable paper to be presented first as my tenure lecture in fall 2000. The methodology would consist of a literature search and review related to integration in my teaching of the Christian perspective into my discipline…. I am very excited about the reading I have begun on being Reformed and on the Reformational worldview….
>
> In conclusion, I believe it is important that the discipline of nursing on Trinity's campus has scholarly representation both on campus and in the larger community. I am pleased to say that I have just published (October 1999) my dissertation work in a refereed nursing journal which acknowledges me as faculty at Trinity Christian College. In addition, I have just completed an invited book chapter on leisure programs for Springer Publishing Company, scheduled for publication in 2000…. If granted this sabbatical, it would be a pleasure for me to extend further the scholarly representation from our nursing department to both the campus and larger community and to continue to role model scholarly endeavors, rather than only nursing practice, to our nursing students.

I was encouraged by the possibility of being granted a sabbatical. I wanted time to process my now bubbling-below-the-surface emotions over Marv's illness. I wanted to be free for awhile from the constant demands of teaching. I wanted, with fewer distractions, to fulfill my dream of completing the scholarly projects.

At the end of the fall semester, I ran into the nursing supervisor of the orthopedic unit coming out of the nurses' station. "How's it going, Lois?" she asked.

"It's going well, Marsha. The students have given their nine o'clock meds, and we even had a few insulins this morning, so several got to give shots. Now they're doing their baths. They're doing fine, but I'm not sure how long I'm going to be able to keep up this pace!"

"I know what you mean. That's why I left teaching. This job is less demanding."

"It's a bummer for older bones." I laughed. "I get off at noon and go straight home to bed. When I get up in the morning, I leave on my electric blanket. All morning I dream of the warm cocoon waiting for me. No one at the college knows I do this. I'm back, bright and perky, for three-thirty meetings. Lucky, I live close." I paused. "Regular massages keep me going, too."

"Good for you. Well, if you aren't back next fall, I'll understand." She smiled.

"Thanks! When I think that only two years ago I went back to the college from a day like this and taught a lab for three hours, I don't know where that stamina came from. I no longer have it. It's up and left."

Marv and I spent Christmas again with Jon and Sheri and our grandchildren in Seattle. Marv had a bit more pep, but still the possibility that his health could deteriorate any day nearly consumed us. And, even though we had promised our kids we'd never spend another Christmas in dreary Seattle like the last one with its constant rainy drizzle, the thought of Marv dying prompted us to do strange things, including Marv going with me to shop for presents—a first.

One afternoon in Seattle I met my sister Rose in Bellevue Square outside Nordstrom. We sat on ice cream chairs. Our usual decaf nonfat mochas helped us ponder life. From nowhere, she asked, "When are you going to retire, Lois?"

"I have no idea, sixty-two or sixty-five. That's a few years off."

"Why wait? What are you waiting for?"

"I don't know. I guess because I don't know what I'd do with all that time. I can't imagine waking up with no place I'd have to go or nothing I'd have to do. It's scary."

Pointing her finger at me, she said, "Lois, trust God."

For the January 2000 Interim back at work, I used what I'd learned in my previous summer's course at Borders to teach Exploring Your Creativity, using Julia Cameron's book, *The Artist's Way*, as a text. My class of nine students shared personal stories of learning flamenco dancing while studying abroad, playing guitar at coffee houses, and snapping photos of strangers in coffee shops. They showed me life could be more than books and studying. They brought me a birthday cake with fifty-eight candles burning and sang "Happy Birthday."

On January 19, the eighth day of the two-week Interim, I fell on the ice on my front porch at seven in the morning getting the paper. Marv was already at work. After bandaging my arm with an Ace wrap, I taught for three hours. No time to go to the doctor.

Life review time. Was I crazy to go to work? Hadn't I always showed up?

Don't nurses always come to work, sick or not?

Everything hurt; I had twisted my body as I fell down. I zigzagged sideways to coddle the pulled muscles in my groin. The next day I announced: "We'll wrap up today, one day early, because I'm having a lot of pain, and like any good nurse, I will finally call the doctor this afternoon." The students, of course, were jubilant. A long weekend for them.

I called the doctor the next morning. The office referred me to the ER where, after lying five hours on a cart in a lone hallway reading a book and feeling famished and thirsty and neglected, I found out my arm was broken. After the ER doctor examined the X-rays, he said: "We'll wrap you now, but you must see an orthopedic doctor in two days for potential casting."

I asked, "Why do I need to wait?"

He said, "You can't be casted until two days after the break."

I said, "It's already been two days."

Disbelief rutted his face. "What do you mean? What took you so long to get here?" He obviously didn't know nurses very well. He could've asked Marv. "Then you must go now. I'll give you directions."

My left arm, wrapped in a bulky dressing, was secured to my body with an array of straps. I slipped the sleeve of my long down winter coat up my right arm and left the ER with the coat draped over my left shoulder, sloshing through the parking lot to my car. I called Marv on my car phone: "Can you meet me at an orthopedic doctor's office? I may need to be casted."

"Casted? Is your arm broken?" I didn't dare try to picture his face. I heard a deep sigh. "Sure, honey. I'm on my way home anyway. Where will you be? Be careful driving one-handed. Roads are slick."

A few days later I came home from my first day of clinical on a psychiatric unit after teetering across slippery sidewalks to the ice-furrowed parking lot. I flopped down at our kitchen bar and, while I was securing my broken arm with Velcro into an immobilizer that I wasn't allowed to wear on the unit, Marv, making dinner at the counter, asked, "How was your first day?"

"Well," I started, "the student group looks fun, the patient mix is going to be a good learning experience—everything from depression, to bipolar disorder, to schizophrenia, and the staff were happy to see me back."

Normally, these are the ingredients for a good clinical experience. But as I finished my declaration, I slumped over the bar and burst into tears.

"What's wrong?" Marv asked, turning from the stove with one hand holding a stirring spoon and the other wearing a glove potholder.

Asking for a tissue, I answered, "Everything was fine—it could not have been better. But I am so tired, so unbelievably tired. And I hurt all…"

"Then quit." He stared directly at me for a quick second and then turned back to take leftovers out of the microwave.

Quit? When I'd worked hard and long to achieve the rank of full professor and get tenured? When I was doing what I liked to do? When I liked the fun I had with students?

I looked at the graying fringe on the neckline of his thick hair. Did he not get it?

Twenty-eight

ON MY WAY

The evening Marv told me to quit I lay back in my blue recliner, placed my pencil over lecture notes I was reviewing, and closed my eyes. Could I really quit working early? At fifty-eight? A year later, while taking my first ever poetry class, I wrote my image of what happened next:

THE WAVE
In my mind I was standing
On the shore of Lake Michigan
Getting my feet wet
Facing the sun on the horizon

Waves lapped my ankles
Suddenly a new wave appeared
Rushing toward me from my right
Washing heavily over my chest
Engulfing me, lingering a moment

Leaving as quickly as it came
Rippling forward to my left
Out to sea
And I was free

I was now free from my unrest that had begun with the family and friend illnesses two years before, and then was capped off with Marv's illness, but I was plain worn out. I had yet to acknowledge I'd been diagnosed with fibromyalgia somewhere during this time. I didn't want to have it, knew of its reputation of belonging to hypochondriacs, so must have decided if I didn't say "hello" to it, it wouldn't be there.

That denial had worked in my head, but not in my body. I had the classic symptoms of fatigue and muscle burning from arms to trunk to legs. That first day on the massage table two and a half years earlier, when I was letting off sparks of energy from red hot muscles, should have alerted me that I needed to listen to my body and slow down.

The Lake Michigan wave that visited me on the evening of my indecision was reassuring. I was certain God had sent it as a sign. I could let go. I could quit early. I could trust Him to help me figure out what to do with the rest of my life.

A few days later, on Wednesday, February 2, 2000, I e-mailed Marianna:

Just had a long conversation with Marv. I have decided to resign. It came to me clearly Monday night that this is enough. Sat on it for two days and we talked about it after clinical today. We meet with our financial advisor tomorrow with her projections of me resigning this year or in two years. So I need to mull over all of this. But it is clear that I have been there, done that. I need to go PLAY.

Feel so, so tearful. Unreal. Like a death. I moseyed down the psych halls today, looking at my reflection, locking in the memory, anywhere I could. There's something so good about nursing, but my body and my mind simply say no more pushing like this. What for? Will cry a little more, then go for a massage. Will find out by Monday if I got my sabbatical. It should work out well for the next person in line—they can get mine. Such an ego thing. So complex.

Thanks for calling yesterday—Marv told me. I was too fatigued and nauseated to respond. Had to do clinical paperwork last night and just sat at the computer totally sick. And it just confirms my decision. No more fatigue. Life is too short.

Oh, my friend, I think only you can understand this awful loss I'm feeling (gut love for it, status, money, sense of identity and belongingness at Trinity…all the positive things,) but also my need to give nursing education up after twenty years. The good thing is, I can pick nursing up in another form if I ever wish. Leaving now for two-hour massage. Lois

I resigned the next week, effective at the end of the semester. I bought several dozen miniature Danish pastries and put them out on a table in our nursing office for the students and faculty. Next to the large boxes, I posted a sign, quoting Browning: "Grow old along with me, the best is yet to be…." As the nursing faculty arrived for work and students dropped in, laden with coats and books, there were surprised hugs, "Congratulations," and comments of "How very nice for you!"

Spring semester, I tried to make a memory of each moment of teaching my mental health nursing course for the last time. In the classroom, I ad-libbed from typed lecture notes that I distributed. I had never liked formal lecturing or being tied to lecture notes. I'd much rather—as students said in my evaluations—"tell stories." I knew they were "clinical anecdotes" and trusted my administrative evaluators would understand. From my years in teaching, I could pull up a story in seconds that pertained to any of the course content. If I pictured a bedside, a dayroom, or a nurses' station, images of patients popped into my mind. And the students and I sang what I called my theme hymn for the course: "Lead Me, Guide Me." I needed God's guidance myself, but also told students to hum this on their first jobs when they were feeling alone.

In clinical, when the students and I walked on the unit the second day, we faced an older unshaven, uncombed male patient sitting in a vinyl easy chair near the entry. He joked, "Here you are again, with your ducklings following you." I'd never thought of my students as ducks, but the image made me smile. And made me wonder how it would feel not to have any flocks following me after nearly twenty years. Lonely? Free? A little of both? The latter.

On one of the last days of clinical, I did my usual thing and sat down at a table in the dayroom. A female patient around forty joined me. Her eyes were red and puffy, her hair straight and stringy. I greeted her, told her who I was, and handed her a stack of Xeroxed pages from a new coloring book. She picked out a dog picture and started shading it in browns. I picked out a train conductor—I wanted to take my last coloring project home and put it on the fridge next to my grandchildren's—and began striping his costume in black and white. The woman suddenly stopped and looked at me. "I'm afraid my kids are going to throw me out. They say I'm acting crazy…. They don't understand I have these times when I feel I need to run away."

"Run away?" I asked. I certainly understood. And again felt grateful for how my life had turned out.

As the seven-week class came to a close, I began to feel the way the people living with a long-term mental illness must have felt on a teaching video I showed during the module on schizophrenia. In *We're On Our Way*, narrated by Burt Lancaster and produced by the Eldan Company, persons living with a long-term mental illness talked about their hopes for the future, grabbed arms and swayed and sang: "We're on our way and we won't turn back...." When the video came to the point of the patients singing, I started to sing along and motioned, like a choir director, to have my class sing with me. Singing along put huge smiles on our faces and made us happy to see that these people could feel hope in what appeared to be hopeless situations.

I, too, was on my way. Somewhere. And I wouldn't be turning back.

Trying to make a point one day, I hit my right hand against my breastbone. Clink, jingle. Students' eyes popped. Bewildered, I asked, "What was that?" and smashed my hand against my chest again. Another jingle. Burning red, I giggled. "Oh no, it's my keys. I have no pockets today for my office keys."

The students didn't forget. A few weeks later at a luncheon before graduation, the class gave me a gift certificate to Victoria's Secret.

And, at our annual end-of-year faculty-student-staff party to which I'd worn purple, broadcasting my impending status as an old woman who could wear purple (and an apricot, indigo, or emerald hat if I wanted), the students flooded me with purple presents, including lavender pens and an amethyst notebook to honor my newly announced hope of becoming a writer.

The night before graduation, I attended the baccalaureate chapel, a service planned and carried out by the graduating seniors for their family and friends. These programs made my eyes mist as I'd see the graduates dressed up and taking charge. As I sat in the church waiting for this chapel to start, I remembered being invited back in 1992, the year after I'd left for the research position, to address the students at their pre-chapel pinning ceremony in this same church. I had titled my speech "Making a Difference." I pictured my former students sitting in front of me and making them repeat with me, "If a patient's S-C-A is less than his T-S-C-D, he will have an S-C-D," a phrase I'd taught the students two years earlier that they now half-shouted, smiling and in crescendo, with me. The entire audience giggled when the point was being made that students would remember what they had learned at Trinity forever.

I also remembered the chapel at the end of the first year I'd come back: 1997. I liked to chat with and question family members afterwards. On that night, I was among the last to leave the social hour in the church. One older couple remained in the church's foyer. I caught up to them with my first question. "Where are you from?"

"Iowa."

"Which graduate are you here for?"

"Sarah Van Dyke."

"Really? She's one of my students. I just had her in psych. I didn't know she was from Iowa."

"Yes, we're from the Pella/Peoria area."

"You're kidding. My dad was a minister in Peoria when I was born. In 1942." The woman's eyes widened. "Who was your dad?"

"Dewey Hoitenga."

Words bubbled out of her mouth. "Then you must be Lois. I lived with your folks when your mother had to go to bed the last months of her pregnancy. I stayed on after you were born, but your folks moved when you were about a year old. You may have heard of me. Your older brother and sisters called me Aunt Clara."

I was floored. Of course, I had heard of an "Aunt Clara" who ran the household, during my mother's toxemia that almost led to my folks' termination of the pregnancy, the "auntie" my grandma referred to in her poem to my mother when I was born. And now I'd finally met her.

The amused "Mr. Clara" chimed in, "We used to take you on our dates. I'd come to the parsonage to pick up Clara, and your mother would hold you out under your arms and say, 'Here, take Lois along.'"

Aunt Clara piped in, "I changed many of your diapers," and laughed.

The next day, before graduation, I was passing the bathroom in the church when I heard a giggly voice say, "Did you know Sarah's grandma changed Dr. Roelofs' diapers?" Judging by the howling that followed, I pictured our seniors doing a last-minute fluff of their hair enjoying the dirty diaper gossip of the day.

I'd had many of these heartwarming serendipitous encounters at Trinity—encounters I knew were providential. I would miss them—having colleagues, students, and staff reach out when I didn't know I needed them; connecting with parents on campus for visit days; meeting students related to my childhood acquaintances in Iowa, New Jersey, New York, Indiana, Michigan.

Now, in the faculty gowning room, I was slipping on my University of Illinois flame red regalia, with its royal-blue, four-pointed, velvet tam, thinking it would be the last time I would wear it, when the dean sidled up to me. "I'll signal you when it's time for your speech."

"What speech?" I asked.

He said I'd have a chance to say a few words to respond to the announcement of my "professor emerita" status.

I hadn't even known I was eligible for emerita status. With my ongoing fatigue, I'd been oblivious to most things other than mindfully making every last clinical and classroom minute count. I wouldn't have to stash my regalia in mothballs; I'd be invited back to process in future convocations and graduations for the rest of my life.

Had I known I was being given the award, I would've wanted Marv to come. His lung and liver lesions were stable. In fact, doctors now said they might have always been there. And his energy level was almost back to normal; he was home draining and cleaning his koi pond with its layered stone waterfall. Afterwards, he would hoe and plant the surrounding bed of hostas, prairie grass, and yellow daffodils. Soon we'd be sitting on the deck on summer evenings watching the bright orange koi glide through the tumble of water.

I clasped my arms in front of me, bunching up the poofy gathered sleeves of my regalia, and tried to think up something to say. My mind became as blank as a newly erased blackboard. I, the woman who could adlib three, or thirty, reasons for anything, couldn't think of one single thing I'd like to say to the students and their families and friends, even though I was certain there were important things I would've wanted to say.

When the president handed me the plaque honoring my "professor emerita of nursing" status, our nursing students, wearing royal blue robes and mortarboards, jumped up among the sea of people seated in the large church, broke into smiles, and clapped. Focusing on their fun faces, it was my turn to tear up. I forgot any phrases I'd tried to formulate. I simply said, "I thank you for teaching me more than I ever taught you."

At home, I placed my plaque on the black wrought-iron picnic table on the deck and called Marv up from the yard to see it. "Congratulations," he said with a wide "I'm happy for you" grin, then hugged me tight with his warm earth-smelling arms and hands.

Sinking my worn out but contented self into bed that night, I thought of my students everywhere—two or three, to my surprise, happily working in research positions. I reread the stirring entries in the journal the seniors in my mental health nursing course had given me. I was filled with joy as I pictured them as new grads in their first jobs running up and down hospital hallways, probably on the night shift, carrying out my mission of caring for all the Sadie Tomczyks in this world.